Swine disorders guide

For this English edition:
Swine disorders guide

Plaza Antonio Beltrán Martínez nº 1, planta 8 - letra I
(Centro empresarial El Trovador)
50002 Zaragoza - Spain

First printing: May 2014

ISBN: 978-84-941975-8-1
D.L.: Z 372-2014

Design, layout and printing:
Servet editorial - Grupo Asís Biomedia, S.L.
www.grupoasis.com
info@grupoasis.com

Warning:
Veterinary science is constantly evolving, as are pharmacology and the other sciences. Inevitably, it is therefore the responsibility of the veterinary clinician to determine and verify the dosage, the method of administration, the duration of treatment and any possible contraindications to the treatments given to each individual patient, based on his or her professional experience. Neither the publisher nor the author can be held liable for any damage or harm caused to people, animals or properties resulting from the correct or incorrect application of the information contained in this book.

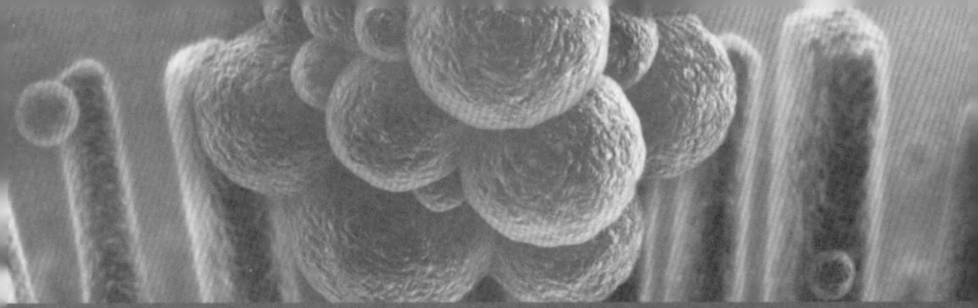

Swine disorders guide

JOHN CARR

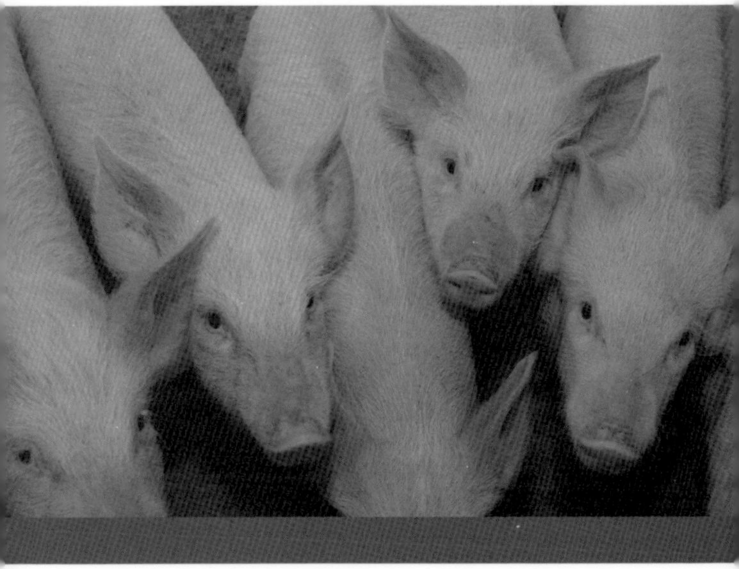

SERVET

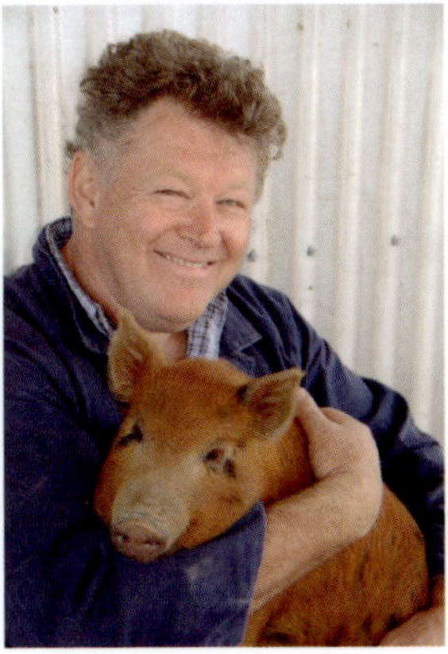

Author

Dr. John Carr

BVSc PhD DPM DiplECPHM MRCVS

John started learning the ropes about pigs at the age of 11. He qualified as a veterinarian in 1982 by the University of Liverpool. After 5 years in general practice he returned to university to complete a Leverhulme residency in pigs and a PhD in urinary tract problems of pigs at Liverpool, where he specialised in microbiology and pathology. He has taught production medicine to veterinarians and farmers throughout the world through positions at several universities in the UK -Liverpool and Royal Veterinary College, London, and in the US -North Carolina and Iowa State- and in Western Australia at Murdoch.

John runs a consultancy practice with clients in North America, Europe, Asia, Australia and Africa. John specialises in maintaining the health of pigs through promoting excellence in stockmanship and production practices while controlling the cost of production. He has published several books and more than 200 refereed and non refereed articles.

http://www.carrsconsulting.com

Preface

Welcome to the book "*Swine disorders guide*". We hope you enjoy the booklet which is aimed to enhance the welfare, wellbeing and productivity of pigs under our care. The pig industry is always improving and the introduction of hyperprolific sows, weaning over 12 piglets and 100 kg per batch farrowing place, is a tremendous improvement. The pig is a great athlete in grow/finish and ensuring that feed is used appropriately is an essential component of profitable pig production. The aim of the booklet is to provide quick, easy and visual guides to the major components to enhance production. Combined with "*The basic stockmanship guide: Pigs, Hogs and Swine*", we hope the booklets encourage debate and discussion within the whole farm team.

We would recommend you have two booklets! One in the pocket, the other in the farm office.

Enjoy.

Dr. John Carr
March 2014

TABLE OF CONTENTS

Conversion table

Distance			
1 inch	2.54 centimetres	1 millimetre	0.03937 inch
1 foot	0.3048 metres	1 centimetre	0.3937 inch
1 yard	0.9144 metres	1 metre	1.094 yards
1 mile	1.6093 kilometres	1 kilometre	0.6214 mile
1 nautical mile	1.8532 kilometres	1 kilometre	1.539 nautical miles
Surface or area			
1 square inch	6.4516 square cm	1 square cm	0.1550 square inch
1 square foot	0.0929 square m	1 square metre	10.76 square feet
1 square yard	0.8361 square m	1 hectare	2.4711 acres
1 acre	0.4047 hectares		
1 square mile	259.0 hectares		
Volume/capacity			
1 cubic inch	16.387 cubic cm	1 cubic cm	0.061 cubic inch
1 cubic foot	0.0283 cubic m	1 cubic decimetre	0.035 cubic foot
1 cubic yard	0.7646 cubic m	1 cubic metre	1.308 cubic yards
Measures			
Imperial		US	
1 pint	0.5506 litre	1 pint	0.473 litres
1 quart	1.136 litres	1 quart	0.9463 litres
1 gallon	4.546 litres	1 gallon	3.785 litres
1 bushel	26.369 litres	1 bushel	35.24 litres
Weight			
1 ounce	28.35 grams	1 gram	0.035 ounce
1 pound	453.59 grams	1 kilogram	2.205 pounds
1 hundred weight	45.36 kilograms	1 tonne	0.984 ton
1 ton	1.016 tonnes	1 bushel (eg corn)	56 lbs (25.4 kg)
Temperature			
º Celsius = [(F-32) x 5)]/9		º Fahrenheit = [(C x 9)/5+32)]	
Energy			
1 joule	0.239 calories	1 calorie	4.184 joules

1

Reproduction of the pig

Enhancing litter size

Age of gilt at first mating	Gilts should be 210 days.
Weight of gilt at first mating	130-140 kg.
Condition of gilt at first mating	20 mm backfat. Feed young gilts well to build up body condition.
Which oestrus in the gilt	Ideally after 2nd oestrus. Note that it is essential to meet batch breeding targets. Mark gilts in each week with a different colour.
Nutrition of gilt from 95 kg	Ad lib feeding up to first mating. Note that the floor feeding may not provide all gilts in the group with ad lib feeding.
Gestation feeding the pregnant gilt	Limit to a condition score of 3.5, or this will create a second litter size drop.
Maximising lactation feed intake	10 kg by day 18 of lactation. Ensure water supply is excellent. Ensure farrowing room is cool enough.
Weaning-to-service	Maximise weaning-to-service increase protein, i.e. fish meal. Possibly keep the sow in the crate and move the piglets and then feed another lactation feed. Do not feed in the morning, move and feed in the evening.
Post-service feeding	Controversial. The standard advice is 2.5 kg, 14 % protein, 18 MJ, 1 % lysine for the first 14 days. May be more critical –first 72 hours post-service.
Feed quality	Mycotoxins can reduce litter size –increase mummified foetuses.
Vitamin A injectable	1 million units at time of weaning in sows and 5 days prior to service in gilts (15 days after last recorded heat). Retinol palmitate used.

Continued ▸

Lactation length	Greater than 17 days[1].
Parity	Minimise drop-outs from herd to 10 % per parity. Parity 3-5 most productive. Replacement rate needs careful management. Ensure herd parity is correct.
Genetics	Heterosis on maternal side may account for 1 pig per litter. Sows with large litters will tend to produce large litters next time. Specific-Meishan effects.
Diseases	Ensure vaccination against *Parvovirus* is up-to-date. Swine Influenza reduces litter size. Teschoviruses, PCV2 and and other viruses may reduce total born piglets, decrease livebirths and increase mummified foetuses and stillbirths.
Movement/stress	Move at service or at 28 days once confirmed pregnant. Implantation occurs at approximately 14 days. Do not move or stress females from 7 to 21 days.
Air quality	Air temperature: 16-18 °C. No draughts.
Boar fertility	Note Swine Influenza and heat stress (infection and environment).
Mating management	Cross-serving. Two services. Natural service and AI[2]. Good, polite stockpeople.
Light patterns	The service area in particular needs to be well lit and have a 16 hours on and 8 hours off on a time clock. 500 lux required.
Maximise gilt litter	To maximise lifetime performance use gilts as foster mothers.
Farrowing management	Reduced stillbirths and accurate stillbirths/pre-weaning mortality.
Post-service environment	Provide quiet post-service management to allow sows to sleep post-mating.

[1] Lactation length in sows. To complete lactation length in piglets (in the European Union, this should be at least 21 days), it is possible to design a cross-fostering programme.

[2] In industrialised production systems, artificial insemination is used for the two services.

The courtship sequence in pigs

Aids in the detection of oestrus

- Have the assistance of a boar, **preferably a mature boar** which is producing a large amount of pheromones (scents) that stimulate the female. He must be trained in the layout of the dry sow house/ gestation area, but must not become too accustomed to the work, or he will only detect the sows´ which waste their feed.
- Oestrus detection should start **three days after weaning and continue three times daily until served and twice daily for the entire duration of pregnancy.**
- **The boar should be presented to the head of the sow or gilt.** Note that this is only stage one of the courtship sequence.
- House sows and gilts no closer than 10 metres from the boars. Ideally the sows and gilts should not be able to see the boars until the time to mate.
- It is essential to have at least 20 minutes a day of boar exposure to induce oestrus. Constant exposure can be detrimental to the length of oestrus exhibited.
- **Heat detection is easier if sows and gilts that do not have boar stimuli (sight, sound or smell) for one hour prior to checking for oestrus.** Gilts only exhibit intense oestrus signs for periods of 7-10 minutes and may take 45 minutes before being able to re-exhibit oestrus.
- **Use another unfamiliar boar if sows or gilts exhibit some of the signs of oestrus, but will not mate.** This is particularly important in a group of gilts where one is detected by one boar but several others in oestrus are missed by the stockperson's enthusiasm for the gilt who exhibits first.

Apply all the principles of stockmanship for heat detection

- Ears, to detect a calling sow.
- Eyes, to detect the restless, nervous sow, which is off her food and has a swollen vulva, which is slightly red.
- Touch, to exhibit back pressure test in the presence of the boar.
- The commonsense, to be quietly patient in observing animals.

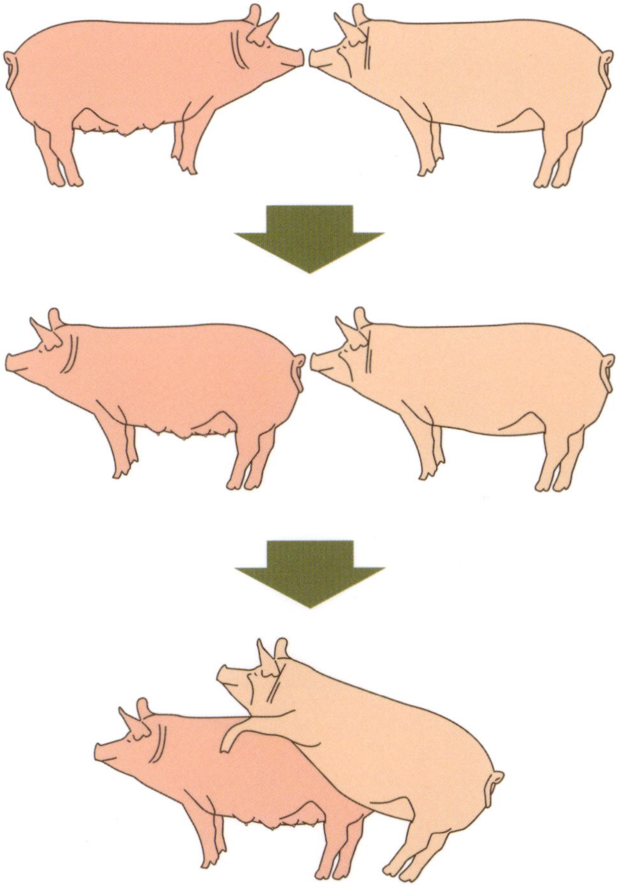

Figure 1. The courtship sequence in pigs.

The signs of oestrus

Pre-oestrus

- ☐ In gilts, the vulva swells, but this sign is not consistent in sows.
- ☐ The vulva becomes congested or red.
- ☐ The udder develops in gilts.
- ☐ The female becomes nervous and easily disturbed.
- ☐ She is ridden by other sows, but does not stand.
- ☐ Vaginal walls become reddened (congested).
- ☐ The clitoris becomes more prominent.
- ☐ Vaginal fluids thicken, produce strands between fingers.

In oestrus

- ☐ The vulva reddening, if present, starts to subside.
- ☐ There is a slight mucous vulvar discharge.
- ☐ The female starts to mount other sows, and if mounted starts to stand.
- ☐ Emits a characteristic high-pitched grunt.
- ☐ Actively seeks boars.
- ☐ Has a decreased appetite.
- ☐ Stands to back pressure, particularly in the presence of a boar.
- ☐ In a Large White, pricks her ears.
- ☐ Rub marks.
- ☐ Has a clean vulva in outdoor units (post service).
- ☐ Rubs and is attracted to stockpeople.
- ☐ Allows coitus.

Reasons for missed heats

Missed heats

Individual variation in intensity of oestrus	• Vulva changes. • Behaviour of sow or gilt.
Unsuitable environment for demonstration of oestrus	• Restricted movement. • Poor facilities –light, floor, etc. • Insufficient boar stimulation. • Distractions.
Inhibition of signs of oestrus	• Lameness. • Illness. • Fear. • Rough inexperienced boar.
Signs of oestrus missed	• Poor records. • Stockperson training. • Boar issues.

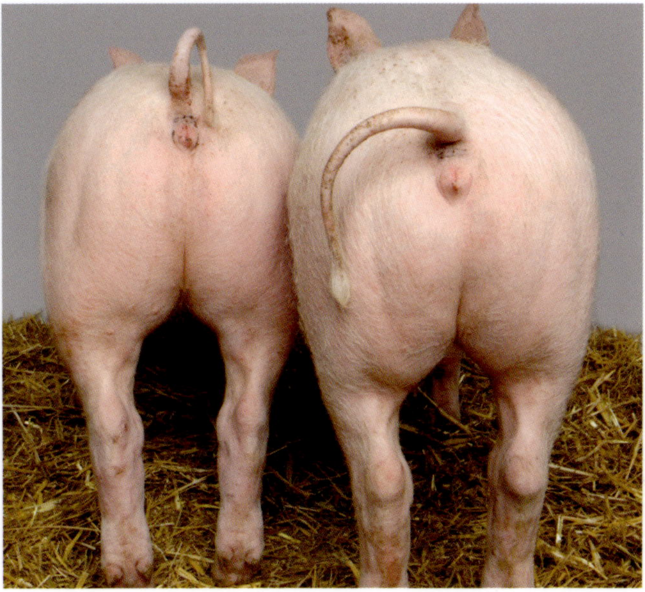

Major reasons for reduction in farrowing rate

REASON	TARGET %
Total returns: • Regular returns 18-24 days post-service. • Irregular returns any other time post-service.	< 10 < 8 < 2
Not pregnant (> 80 days post-service)	0-0.5
Abortion	0.5-1
Culls (pregnant)	< 1
Deaths (pregnant)	< 1
Farrowing rate	**> 87**

Reasons for return

DAYS AFTER SERVICE	REASONS FOR RETURN
0-17	Nymphomaniac. Not in season initially.
18-24	Oestrus.
25-35	Embryonic death. Not in season initially.
36-48	Missed oestrus.
49-80	Pseudo pregnancy, abortion, combination of above.
80+	Combinations of above.

Pregnancy diagnosis

Probe position

Place probe against flank. Aim just behind opposite shoulder and slowly rotate hand backwards.

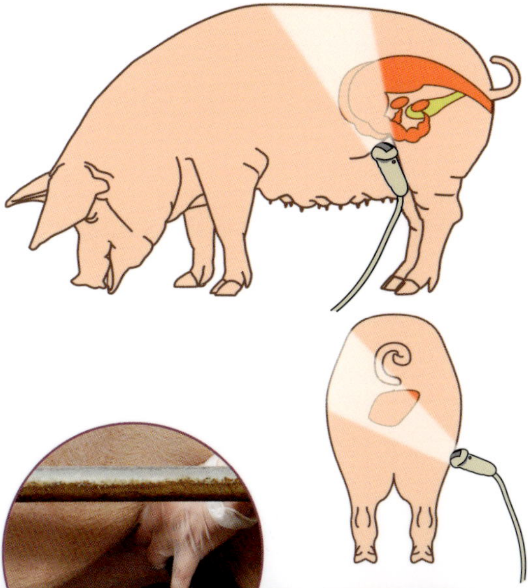

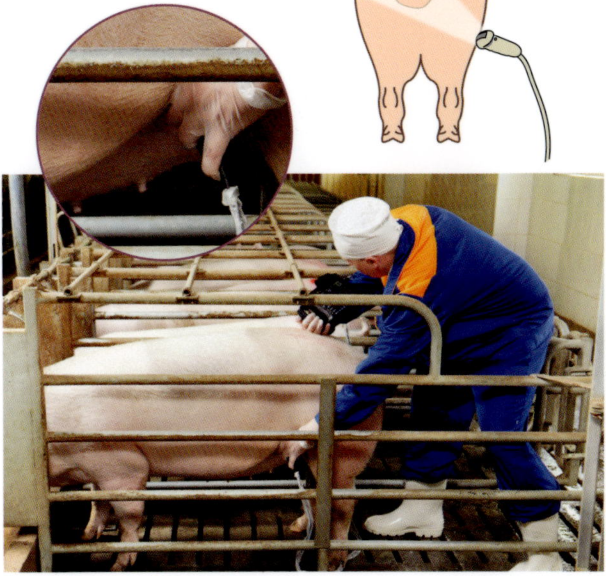

Pregnancy diagnosis

1-115 days	In the presence of the boar.
18-24 days	In the presence of the boar to checking for regular oestrus return.
25-34 days	In the presence of the boar to check for late returns.
28 days	• With the Doppler machine for uterine pulse. • Real time ultrasound.
35 days	With the Doppler and Real time ultrasound for uterine pulse.
8 weeks	• By eye, looking for dropped abdomen. • Any questionable sow, recheck with Doppler for uterine pulse and foetal pulse or real time for foetus.

False positives: false uterine pulse when the sow is coming or in season.
This is why you need two positives (28 and 35 days) to be confident that the sow is pregnant.
A sow which records one negative must be rechecked the following day.
A sow with two negatives must go back to the boar and be rechecked.

- Always check that the Doppler machine is well serviced and has a well-charged battery.
- Regularly re-listen to the teaching tape.
- Use plenty of gel between the head and the sow's body wall.

Result interpretation using a Doppler

RESULT		SIGNIFICANCE
28 days	35 days	
+ve	+ve	Pregnant.
-ve	+ve	Coming into second oestrus return.
+ve	-ve	Embryonic death possibly.
-ve	-ve	Not pregnant.

A sow wrongly believed to be in pig post 35 days costs you around 11.4 pigs sold –1,000 kg pork.

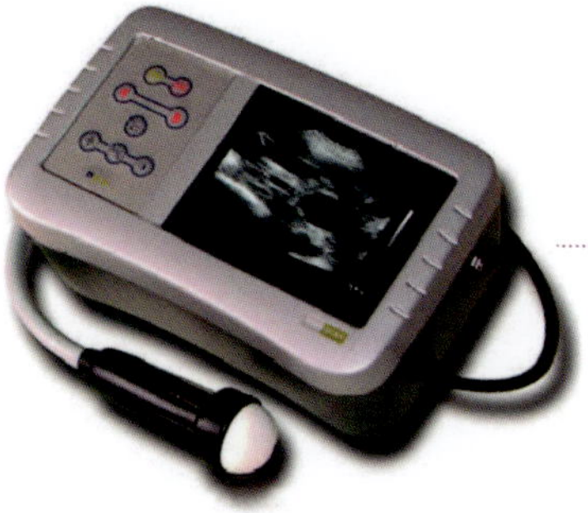

Real-time ultrasound basics

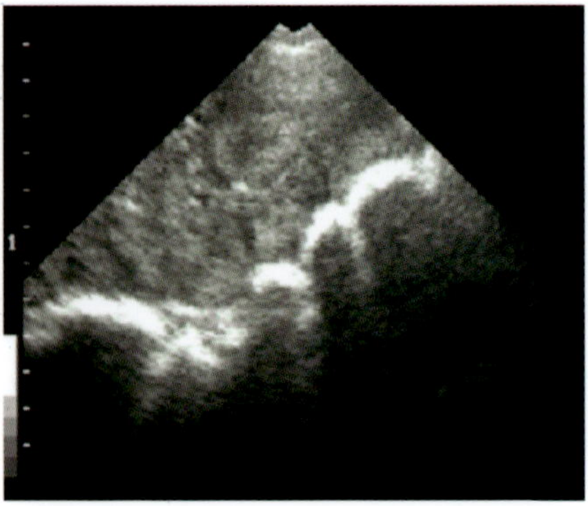

Not pregnant

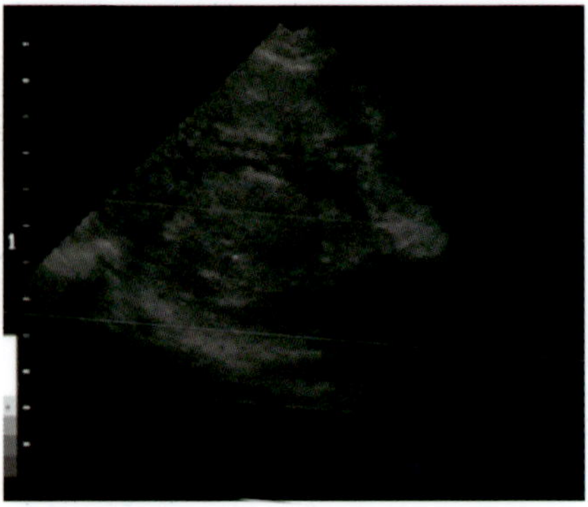

In oestrus

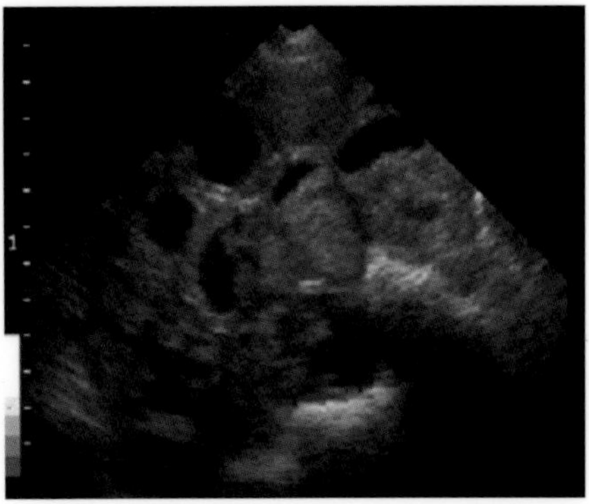

Early pregnancy

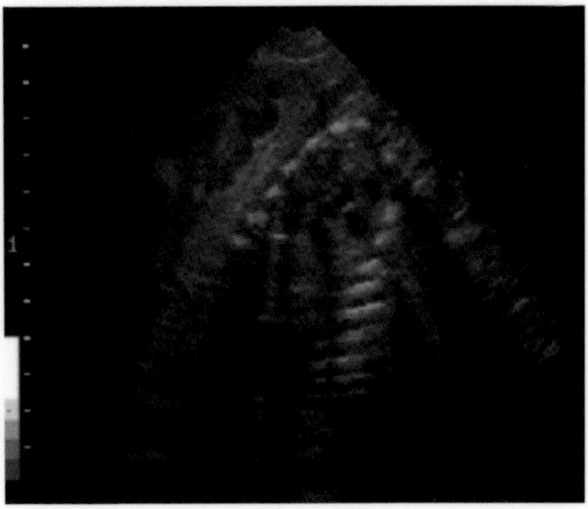

Late pregnancy

Foetal age estimation

The age of a foetus can be estimated using the following formula:

[Crown-to-rump length (mm)/3] + 21 = age in days

Examples

CROWN-TO-RUMP LENGTH (mm)	AGE ESTIMATE (days)
25	29
50	38
75	46
100	54
150	71
200	88
250	104

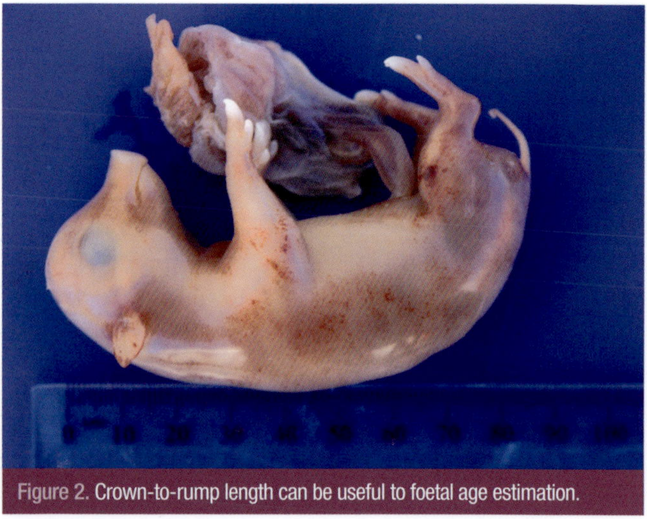

Figure 2. Crown-to-rump length can be useful to foetal age estimation.

Weaning-to-breeding interval

Effect on production targets

Farrowing rate assuming a lactation of more than 18 days

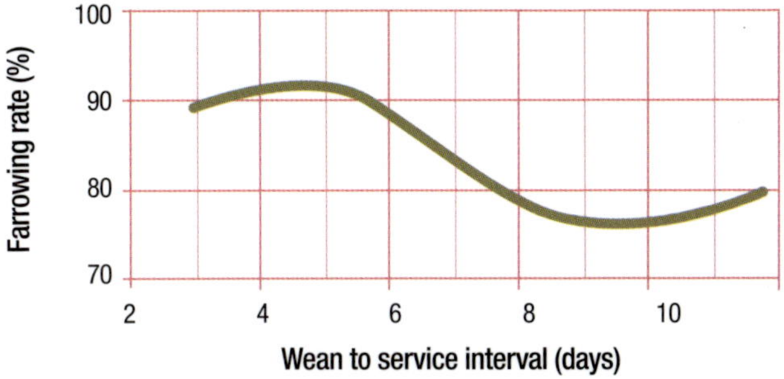

Between 3 and 5 days post-weaning, there is little reduction in farrowing rate. However, the reduction is dramatic between days 7 and 12.

Subsequent litter size assuming a lactation of more than 18 days

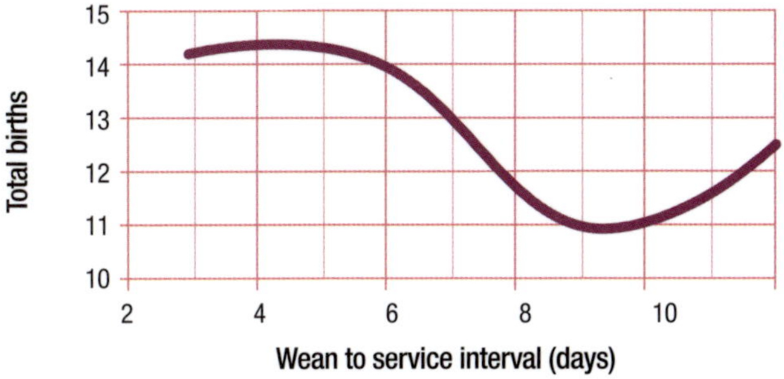

The litter size follows a similar pattern to the farrowing rate.

Factors that reduce the weaning-to-service interval

Lactation feeding	• The aim is to reduce weight loss during lactation. • The sow should eat 10 kg by day 18 of an 18 % protein, 1 % lysine, 9.7 MJ NE (14.5 MJ DE). • Average consumption is required to be over 7 kg per day. Additional chromium may help. Biotin to be at 2.25 μg/kg.
Weaning-to-breeding feeding	• Continue with lactation feed: 4 kg a day to point of service. • Feed once a day. • Ensure that water supply is more than adequate, particularly after breeding, to help prevent cystitis problems.
Day of service to 3 days post-service	• Feed the dry sow with a ration of 1.5 to 2 kg a day. Nevertheless, the sow may not eat much anyway while in oestrus. • Gilts must not be overfed in the immediate period post-breeding as this can affect litter size. Sows are less vulnerable.
3 days post-service-to-farrow	• Follow dry sow feeding routines. First 3-21 days of gestation increasing feed may help placental growth in sows. • Overfeeding in gestation will affect subsequent lactation feed intake.
Boar exposure	• Limited exposure only for the first 2 days post-weaning. • Then 20 minutes a day from day 3 to service. Actual boar contact. • Ideally heat check/stimulate twice or even three times daily. • Remove boar from the sow breeding area, by 10 metres –sight, sound, smell– for one hour before breeding.

Breeding barn environment

Water	Adult sows drink 8 to 12 litres per day. If water is supplied through a nipple drinker, aim to provide 1.5 to 2 litres per minute. If water is supplied via a front water trough, ensure the water is fresh and clean, and refill the trough at least 3 times a day, perhaps providing 5 replenishments in the summer months.
Light and air	16 hours of daylight and 8 hours of dark are ideal. The light intensity required is 500 lux, about the light intensity in your kitchen. Many breeding areas are poorly lit. The breeding area must be draught-free and the sows kept at between 16 and 22 °C. If the temperature exceeds 22 °C, cooling is required.
Floor	The floor in the breeding area must provide good footing and ensure neither the boar nor the sow slips on the floor. The flooring in the sow housing must be non abrasive. In many farms, metal and tops of bolts can come into contact with the sow and can cause abrasions. Any slatted flooring should be pencil-edged. The sows should be provided with 2.7 m^2. Avoid mixing gilts and 1st parity sows with older sows in loose housed accommodation.
Feed	All feed should be fresh and must not contain mycotoxins. Note that this means feed barrows should be protected from the rain and feed bins regularly cleaned. Home mixers should regularly check that their feed supplies the correct mix of ingredients. Feed access, particularly between the weaning and time of breeding, must be optimised. This may be particularly important for gilts and 1st parity sows. Gilts may benefit from a high energy, low protein ration to help put on backfat without a large frame.
Stock	Ensure that the sow/gilt and boars are of the correct size.

If any sign of lameness is detected, you should serve by artificial insemination only.

Seasonal effects on farrowing rate

While the domestication of the pig has reduced seasonal effects more dramatically than in sheep (for example), it is difficult to completely negate nature's demands. From the pig's point of view, it is unwise to become pregnant in the autumn as the litter would be born in the middle of winter and would likely die. The effects of seasonality are less noticeable in sows reared inside, but for outdoor production systems the autumn abortion/summer infertility syndrome is a serious problem.

It is imperative that additional gilts are served to cover these periods of reduced productivity.

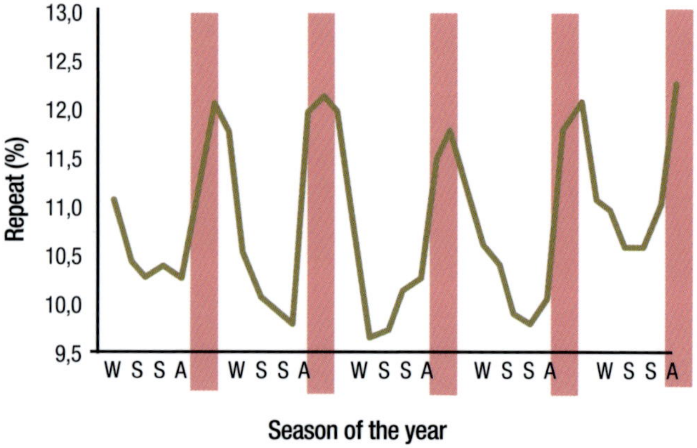

Do not cull sows until the end of the breeding week, or ideally at the point of pregnancy checking. It is essential to breed sufficient to fill the farrowing area and maximise your pig flow.

Second parity litter size drop

A key component to successful pig farming is to maximise the production of the gilt and second litter. These two parities predict the performance of the rest of the sow's life.

It is essential to minimise the loss of gilts becoming 2nd parity sows.

Guide to production expectations

	GILT	2nd PARITY	3-6 PARITIES	7 + PARITIES
Total born	13.9	14.4	14.4	14.6
Born alive	12.9	13.4	13.4	12.9
Stillborn	0.8	0.9	0.9	1.5
Mummified	0.2	0.1	0.1	0.2
Weaned	11.5	12	12	11.5
Farrowing rate %	80	85	87	82
Parity distribution	20	18	60	2

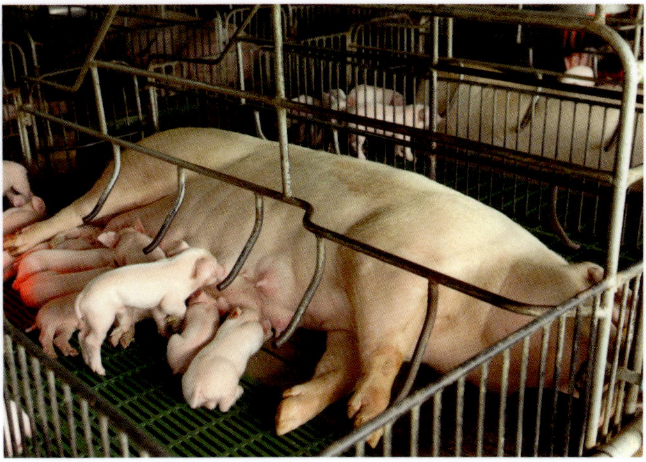

Second parity litter size drop

Cause

Excessive loss of weight and body condition during the first lactation.

How to prevent it

- To ensure long reproductive life, gilts should be in good condition prior to first conception (130 kg, 210 days at 18 mm P_2).
- Introduce a mature boar at 190 days of age. Select gilts that cycle within 14 days of first introduction to a boar. Cull the other gilts.
- Do not over-feed gilts in their first pregnancy as this causes a reduced appetite in lactation.
- Provide a high-energy dry/gestation sow diet, 14 % CP and 0.6 % lysine during pregnancy.
- Gilts should farrow at a body score of 3.5 and appear "plain" and not fat.
- Feed a high-density lactator diet 9.7 NE (14.3 DE) and 1.3 % lysine during lactation. It is possible to enhance intake with 150 g fishmeal top dressed each day.
- Start feeding approximately 2.5 kg per sow on the day of farrowing and build up by increasing to 0.5 kg per sow per day until day 10. Feed ad lib from day 10 onwards. When ad lib feeding is not possible, feed three times per day.
- Ensure gilts eat up to 9 kg a day by day 18 of lactation. Provide sufficient piglets on the gilt to suckle as many teats as possible.
- Wet food boosts the appetite.
- Do not lactate for less than 18 days. Use gilts as nurse sows to extend their lactation length, assuming gilts are eating well.
- Gilts should be provided with 12 pigs after farrowing to encourage feed intake.

Breeding disciplines

The following describes a breeding program for stalled breeding sows. Today is 4 or 5 days post weaning – an ideal breeding day.

Breeding area set up

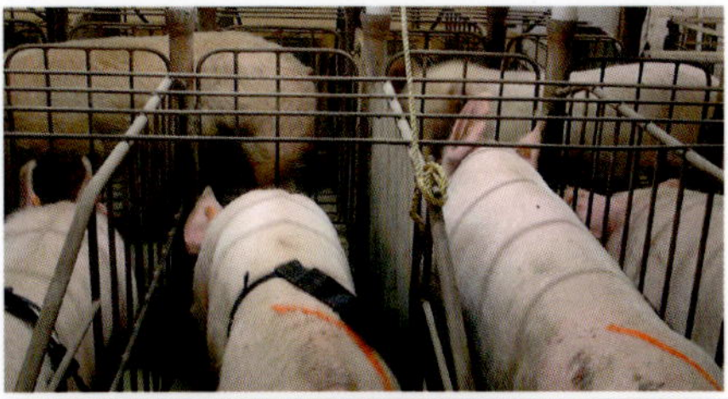

Note stall design incorporates a boar hide. These are set up every third sow.

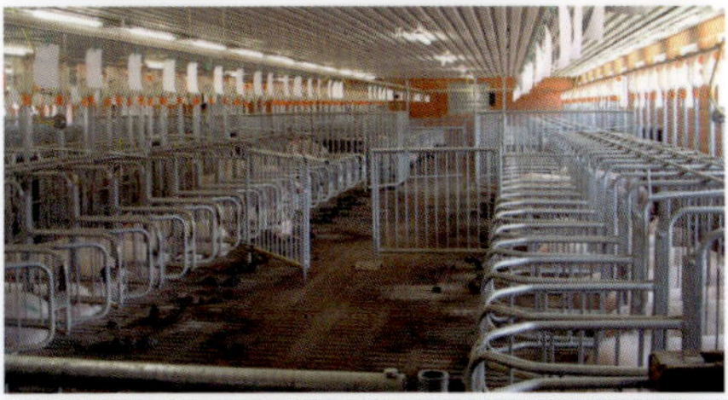

A rear gate which allows easy access to the rear of the sow and her back to aid stimulation.

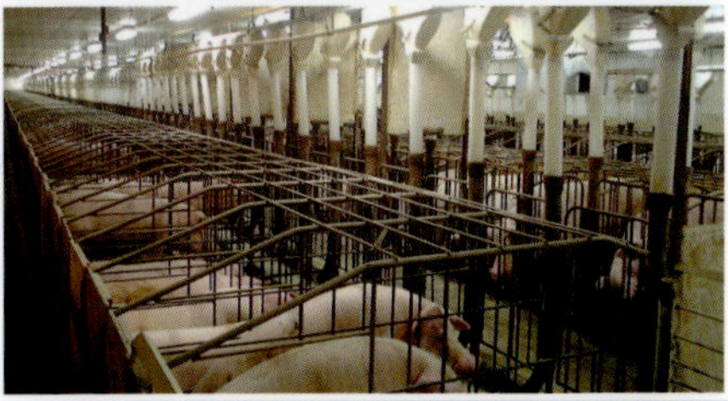

Excellent lighting is essential for good mating.

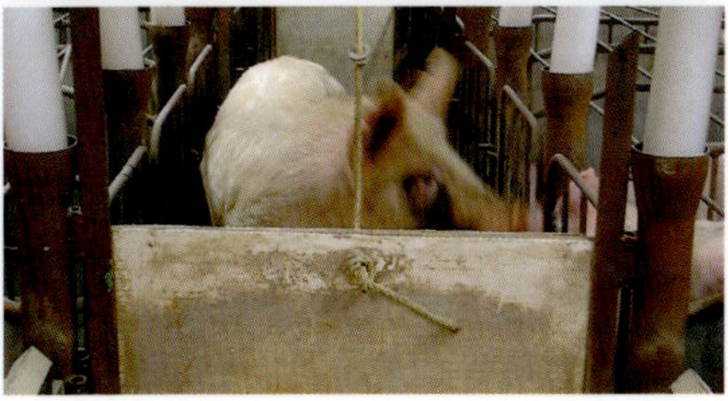

Controlled boar exposure above gates.

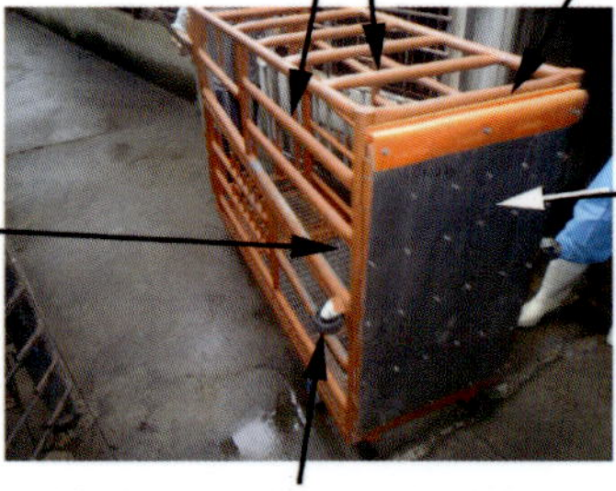

Enclosed crate to stop boar from climbing out
Have handles on front so crate can be pulled
Floor is optional but if boar walking ensure rolling wheels can be locked
Enclosed front reducing exposure to next group of sows
Wheel on sides to keep crate in middle of passageway – 4 would be best

Boar crate which can be moved manually or motorised. Some farms train a boar to walk on a tether and lead.

- Note two separate boars are used to help stimulate the sow and keep both boars interested.
- Ensure that:
  - Boars are housed 10 m or more away from sows.
  - The breeding area is clean and well maintained.
  - There is a safe breeding area for stockpeople.

Breeding routine

Have all the equipment ready.

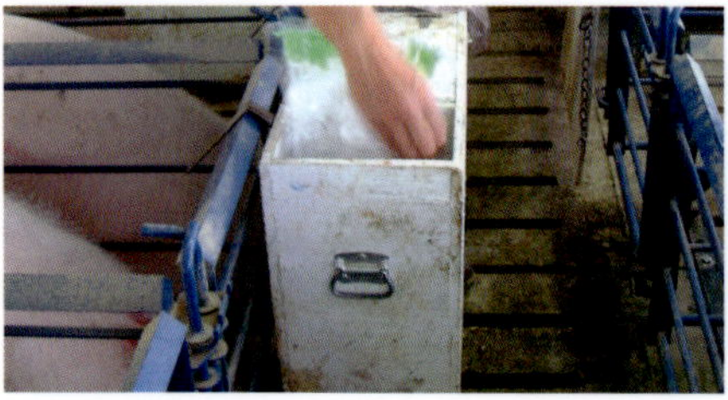

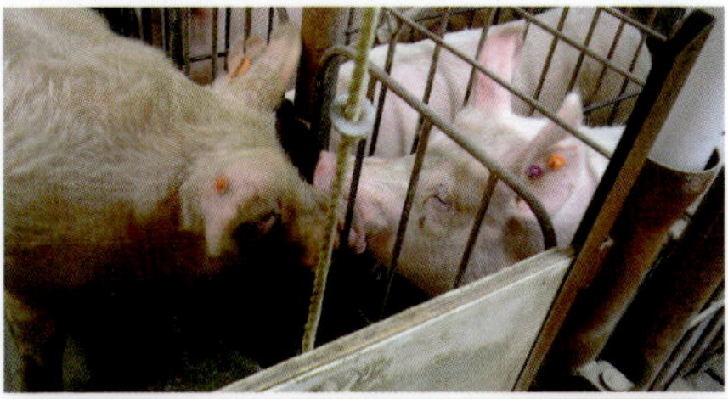

Boar exposed to the sow.

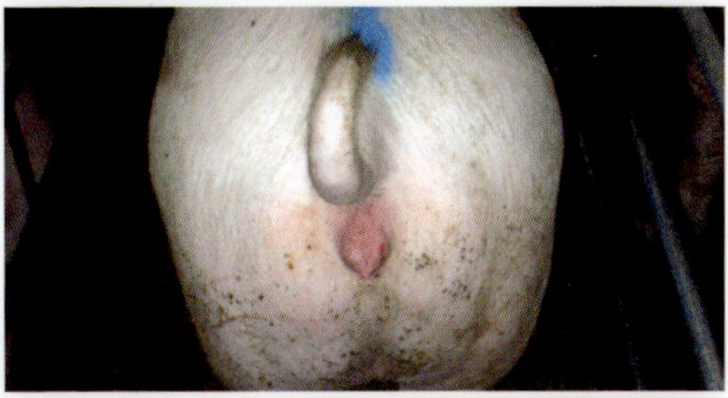

Good signs of oestrus.

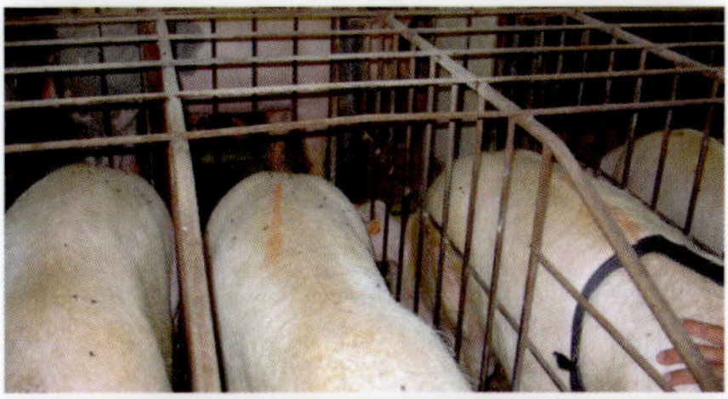

The sow should stand within 30 seconds.

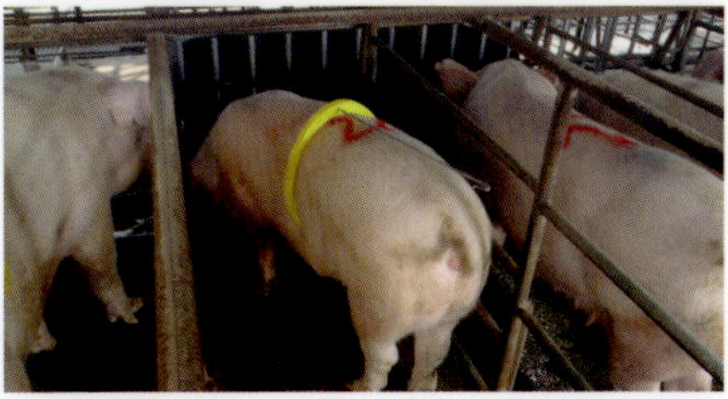

Apply the belt – numerous designs.

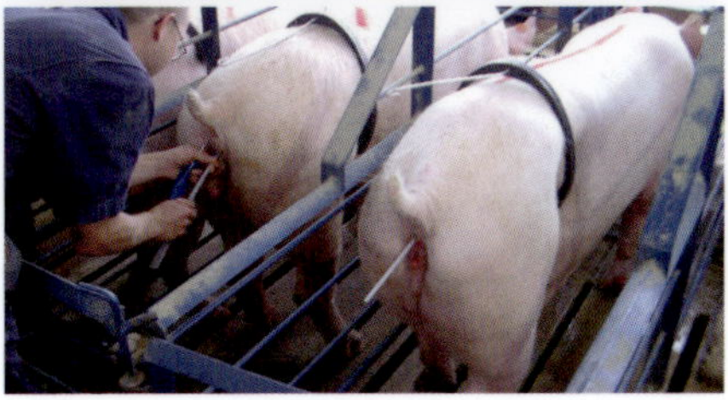

Insert the catheter into the vulva.

Put the semen pack into place at the end of the catheter.

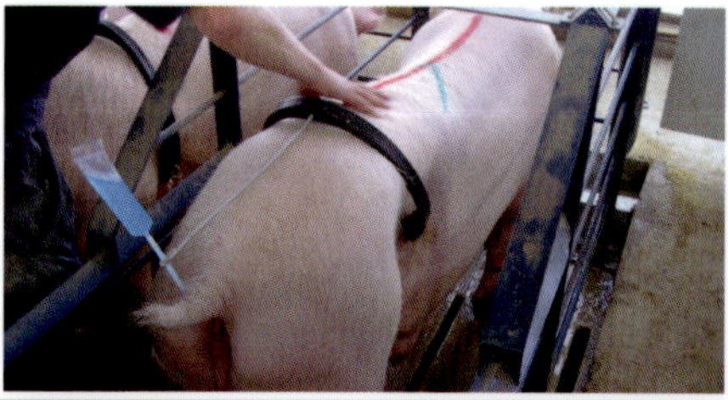

Attach the semen pack to the belt.

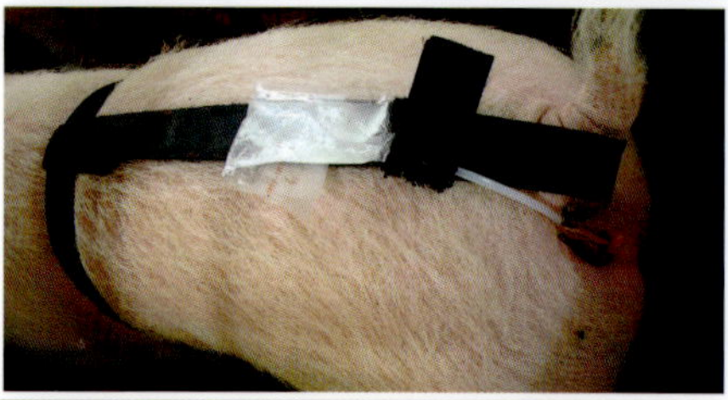

The sow now self serves.

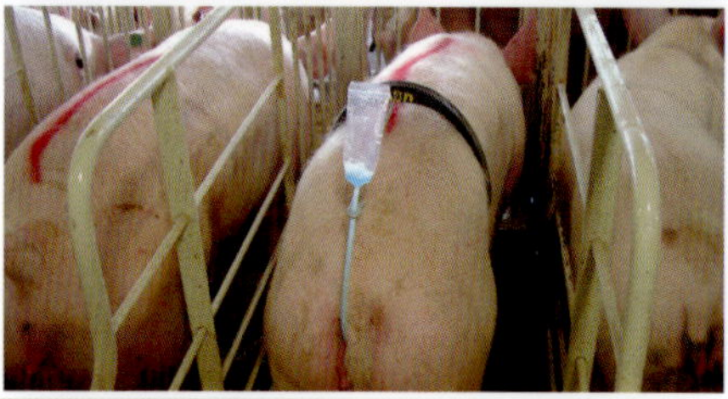

A few sows require extra attention.

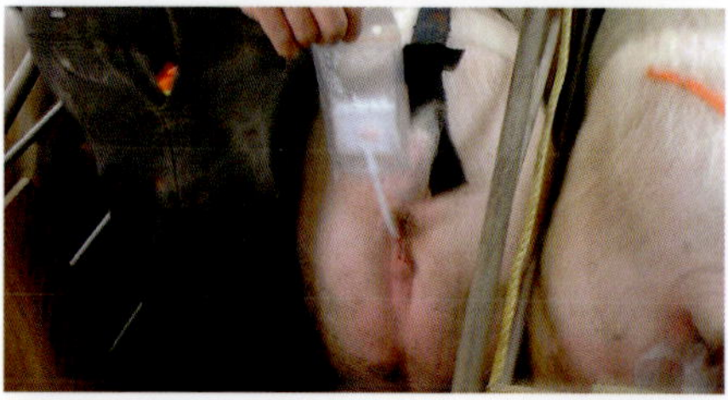

Finish breeding.

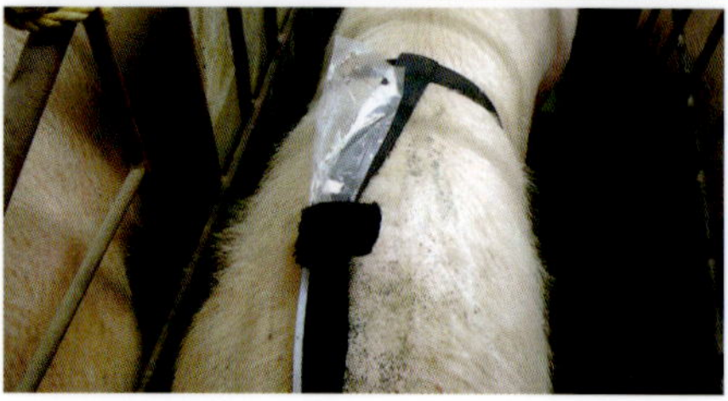

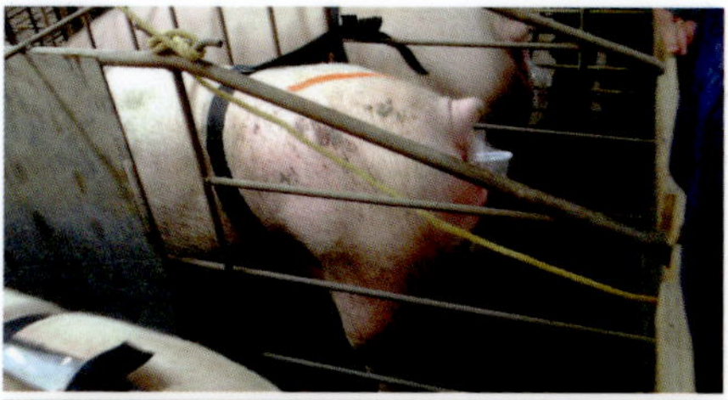

Bend catheter over
into semen pack.

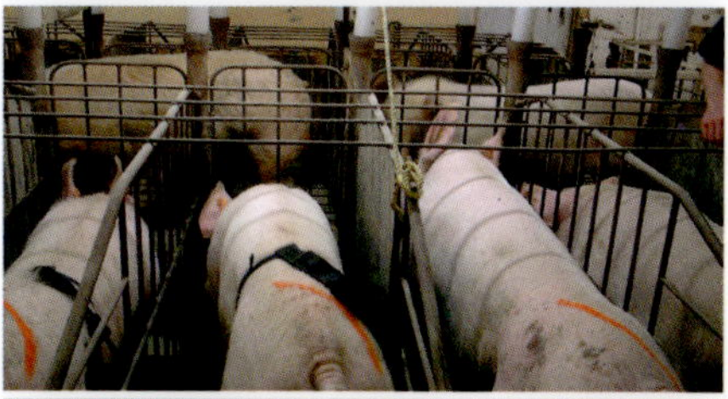

Move boar 1
and introduce boar 2.

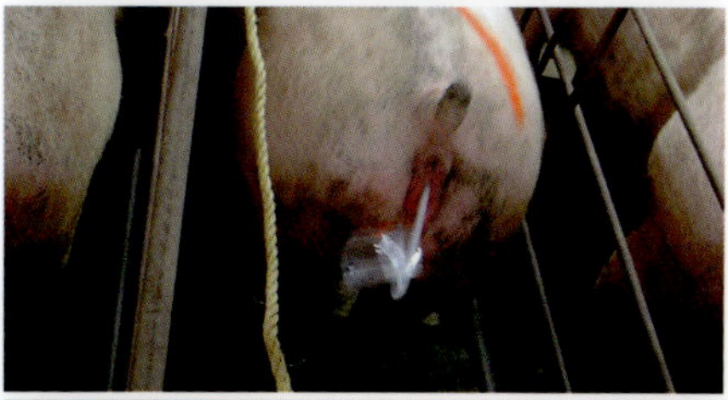

Remove belt.

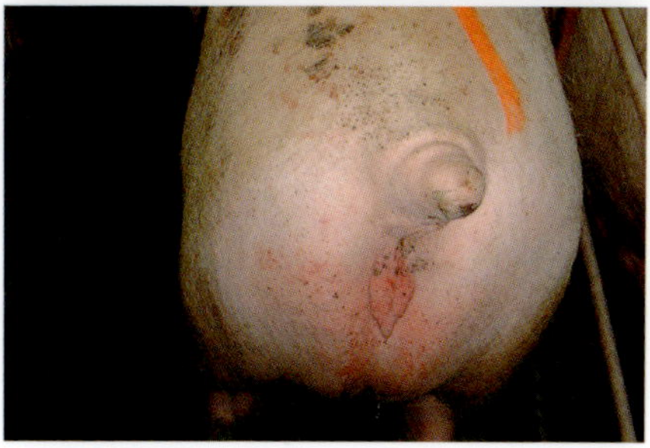

Remove catheter.
Mark sow.

The whole procedure takes two lots of 7 minutes.

Breeding timing for sows weaned on Monday

Double serving

When to mate

The yellow box can be customised.

Day of weaning **Monday**

Days of the week	Tu	W	Th	F	Sa	Su	M	Tu
First oestrus seen	Days since weaning							
	2	3	4	5	6	7	8	9
Wednesday				M	M 0			
Thursday				M	M 0			
Friday				M	M	0		
Saturday					M	M 0		
Sunday						M	M0	
Monday							M 0	
Tuesday								

- When sow likely to be standing (grey box)
- 24 hours before ovulation (pink box)
- 0 Ovulation
- M Mate

Return sows and gilts should be mated naturally (with a boar) at least once.

Single serving for weaned sows

When to mate

The yellow box can be customised.

Day of weaning **Monday**

Days of the week	Tu	W	Th	F	Sa	Su	M	Tu
First oestrus seen	Days since weaning							
	2	3	4	5	6	7	8	9
Wednesday				H	M O			
Thursday				H	M O			
Friday				H	M	O		
Saturday					M	M O		
Sunday						M	MO	
Monday							M O	
Tuesday								

When sow likely to be standing

24 hours before ovulation

O Ovulation

M Mate

H Heat check only

Use double mating programmes for gilts and return sows.

When using single serving, it is recommended to increase the value of the semen in order to improve the FCR and carcase quality.

Note the semen pack contains your future profits – not just water!

Breeding calendar

Breeding date		18 to 24 day repeat			Preg-check (28)		Preg-check (35)		Farrowing (115)	
Jan	1	Jan	19	25	Jan	29	Feb	5	Apr	26
	8		26	1	Feb	5		12	May	3
	15	Feb	2	8		12		19		10
	22		9	15		19		26		17
	29		16	22		26	Mar	5		24
Feb	5		23	1	Mar	5		12		31
	12	Mar	2	8		12		19	Jun	7
	19		9	15		19		26		14
	26		16	22		26	Apr	2		21
Mar	5		23	29	Apr	2		9		28
	12		30	5		9		16	Jul	5
	19	Apr	6	12		16		23		12
	26		13	19		23		30		19
Apr	2		20	26		30	May	7		26
	9		27	3	May	7		14	Aug	2
	16	May	4	10		14		21		9
	23		11	17		21		28		16
	30		18	24		28	Jun	4		23
May	7		25	31	Jun	4		11		30
	14	Jun	1	7		11		18	Sep	6
	21		8	14		18		25		13
	28		15	21		25	Jul	2		20
Jun	4		22	28	Jul	2		9		27
	11		29	5		9		16	Oct	4
	18	Jul	6	12		16		23		11
	25		13	19		23		30		18

Continued ▸

Breeding date		18 to 24 day repeat			Preg-check (28)		Preg-check (35)		Farrowing (115)	
Jul	2		20	26		30	Aug	6		25
	9		27	2	Aug	6		13	Nov	1
	16	Aug	3	9		13		20		8
	23		10	16		20		27		15
	30		17	23		27	Sep	3		22
Aug	6		24	30	Sep	3		10		29
	13		31	6		10		17	Dec	6
	20	Sep	7	13		17		24		13
	27		14	20		24	Oct	1		20
Sep	3		21	27	Oct	1		8		27
	10		28	4		8		15	Jan	3
	17	Oct	5	11		15		22		10
	24		12	18		22		29		17
Oct	1		19	25		29	Nov	5		24
	8		26	1	Nov	5		12		31
	15	Nov	2	8		12		19	Feb	7
	22		9	15		19		26		14
	29		16	22		26	Dec	3		21
Nov	5		23	29	Dec	3		10		28
	12		30	6		10		17	Mar	7
	19	Dec	7	13		17		24		14
	26		14	20		24		31		21
Dec	3		21	27		31	Jan	7		28
	10		28	3	Jan	7		14	Apr	4
	17	Jan	4	10		14		21		11
	24		11	17		21		28		18
	31		18	24		28	Feb	4		25

Pig flow idealised – Space requirements

We can estimate the space requirements for different facilities based on the end product-space allowance for slaughter pig: finishing barn.

Total finishing space available for animals from 30 to 95 kg is 1185.6 m^2.

Animals moved into finishing pens at 30 kg and not moved thereafter. Partially slatted pens.

- Batch time unit: weaning occurs every Monday, batch unit one week.
- Growth curve from 30 to 95 kg.
- Pigs are 10 weeks old at 30 kg.
- Pigs at 110 kg finish being sold at 24 weeks.
- Farm has a 1 week emptying period.
- Therefore, 15 weeks in finishing house.

Weekly grow/finishing space

Space available for batch = 1,185.6 m^2

1,185.6 m^2/15 batchs = 74.1 m^2/batch

Each 110 kg pig requires 0.65 m^2 total area. Therefore:

74.1 m^2/batch/0.65 m^2/pig = 114 pigs/batch

Farm costs

Pigs are sold at 76 kg dead, therefore:

114 pigs/batch x 76 kg = 8664 kg/batch sold

With a cost of 1 price unit per kg (for this farm):

8664 kg sold/batch x 1 price unit/kg = 8664 price units/batch

Post-weaning mortality

The farm has a 5-6 % post-weaning mortality, therefore:

114 pigs/batch + 6 dead pigs/batch = 120 pigs weaned per batch

Weaning space requirements

Pigs weaned at 27 days weight 8 kg and reach 30 kg at the age of 10 weeks. Therefore, 6 weeks of weaner accommodation is required.

Half of the post-weaning mortality occurs in the weaner space i.e. 3 %. Therefore, 117 pigs move into the grow/finish space.

A 30 kg pig requires 0.30 m^2, therefore, the weekly weaner space is:

117 pigs/batch x 0.3 m^2/pig = 35.1 m^2/batch

The weaning period lasts 6 weeks, therefore the total weaner space required is:

6 weeks x 35.1 m^2/batch = 210.6 m^2

Farrowing rate requirements

If 12 piglets are weaned per batch farrowing place per batch, and 120 pigs are weaned every batch, therefore 10 places are required per batch:

120 pigs/batch/12 pigs/farrowing place = 10 places/batch

27 days weaning is a 5 week turnaround, therefore 50 places in 5 rooms/areas of 10 are needed to allow for all-in/all-out.

Number of sows to serve per batch

The number of sows to serve per week should be a minimum of 12.

Sows to serve	Farrowing rate	Farrow per batch
10	100	10
11	> 91	10
12	> 83	10
13	> 77	10

The aim is to create batches of animals moving all-in/all-out through a farming system running 365 days a year, and therefore on a one batch weaning system, 52 batches per year.

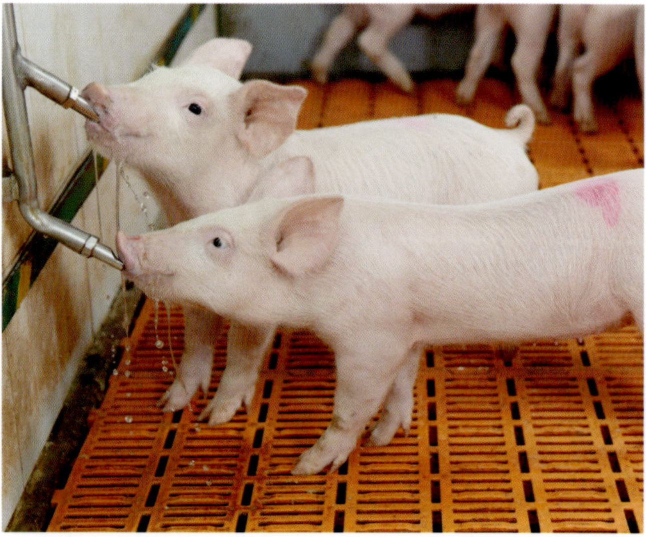

Notes

Pig flow

18 gilt pool 95 kg to service.

12 sows a batch to serve.

10 sows a batch to farrow.

96 kg to wean.

8,664 kg a batch to sell.

450,528 kg paid for annually.

5,928 pigs sold annually.

....

.... gilt pool 95 kg to service.

.... sows a batch to serve.

.... sows a batch to farrow.

.... kg to wean.

.... kg a batch to sell.

.... kg paid for annually.

.... pigs sold annually.

....

.... gilt pool 95 kg to service.

.... sows a batch to serve.

.... sows a batch to farrow.

.... kg to wean.

.... kg a batch to sell.

.... kg paid for annually.

.... pigs sold annually.

Notes

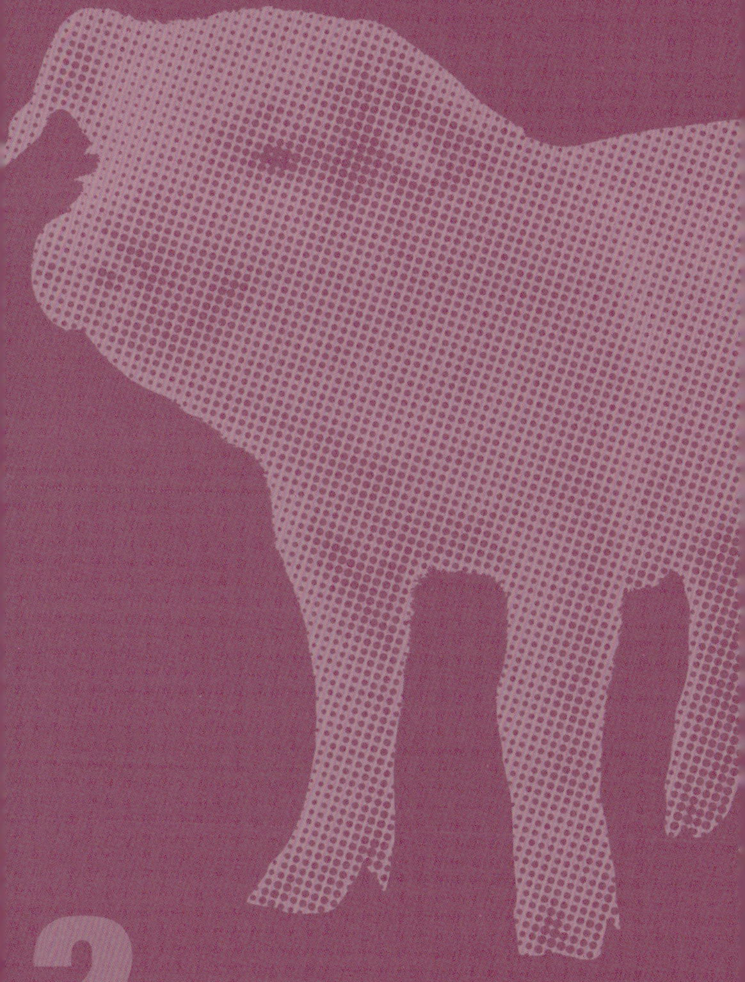

2 Disorders of the pig

Clinical signs for stockpeople

Know what is normal about your pigs – if you don't know what is normal how can you recognise abnormal?

Before entering the pen

Look	Pig not eating	Pigs generally love food and a change in their eating patterns should always be a cause of further investigation.
	Change in behaviour	Depending on the group size pig's individual behaviours may be known or the group has its own behaviour patterns.
		Ideally the stockperson will know all the pigs personally, however, even in a large group; individual pigs tend to stand out, whereas the mass, sadly are unknown. The pigs that do standout are the extremes – the top social order pigs, the lower social pigs and perhaps a few others who have unusual body markings – wolf pig, leopard spotted etc.
	Group behaviours	
	Lying patterns	Try to observe the known pigs and note their lying patterns and position within the group. A sow standing at 14.00 in the afternoon, while all her companions are asleep may be in oestrus. She is exhibiting an unusual behaviour.
	Individual being different	Look for pigs who are separate from the group.
		Note groups of pigs gathered around a drinker or a feeder.

Continued ▸

Listen	Note noises coughing or sneezing	On entry to the room notice the sounds of greeting made by the pigs. Pigs with swine influenza are often very quiet and reluctant to get up as you enter. Well managed pigs should be pleased to see you.
		As the pigs move around, note any coughing or sneezing.
Smell	Become familiar with the normal body odours of pigs. Swine dysentery and swine fever may cause malodorous smells.	

Enter the pen and walk the pigs – in their pen

Look	Look for the individuals, give them memorable names.	
	Movement	Ensure all the pigs get up.
		Note pigs can be stiff or rising, but within 5 to 10 strides the stiffness should walk off.
		Walk over to any pigs who fail to rise or walk off any stiffness.
	Urination	When pigs rise, particularly in the morning, they will urinate within 5 minutes. Note the colour of the urine and the posture of the pig urinating.
	Blood	Look for any blood on the floor or walls.
	Floor	Look at the floor for the consistency of the stools.
Listen	As the pigs move around note any coughing or sneezing.	
Smell	Smell the air – if a pig has died the first indication may be a smell.	

Individual

This includes any pig placed in a compromised/hospital pen.

Pigs housed in small numbers should all be given names. This should include artificial insemination centres and adults on farms of less than 50 sows.

Know	Behaviour	Know the pig's normal behaviour and note any sudden or progressive change in behaviour.
	Feed	Know what food the pig likes and dislikes.
	Reproduction	Know what stage of reproduction the pig is at and note if the expected oestrus behaviour patterns fails to materialise.
		Note changes in males (even when castrated) can occur in the presence of receptive females.
Look	Changes in behaviour – aggressive/less aggressive.	
	Changes in head/ear posture.	
	Changes in eye's brightness.	
	Change in skin colour or hair position.	
	Locomotor changes – reluctance to get up, do normal tricks.	
	Dirty anal/tail area – diarrhoea.	
	Changes in the stools.	
	Signs of vomit.	
Listen	Coughing, sneezing, wheezing and breathing depth.	
Feel	Presence of a lump – may be felt rather than seen.	

Once you have identified that there may be a problem, examine the pig in more detail.

A brief clinical key
What is the major clinical sign?

MAIN CLINICAL SIGN	Causative disorders/agents
Abortions	• Abortion in the sow • Leptospirosis • Pseudorabies – Aujeszky's disease • African swine fever • Classical swine fever • PRRS • Pyrexia • SIV • Erysipelas
Abscess	• *Trueperella pyogenes* • *Actinobacillus pleuropneumoniae* 3 • Streptococci infections
Anaemia	• Iron deficiency • Gastric ulceration • Ileitis – PIA • Swine dysentery • *Mycoplasma suis*
Breathing – heave line	• Glässer's • *Mycoplasma hyopneumoniae* – Enzootic pneumonia – PRDC • *Pasteurella/Streptococcus* pneumonia • PMWS • *Salmonella*
Breathing deep	• APP – *Actinobacillus pleuropneumoniae* • Lice • *Pasteurella/Streptococcus* pneumonia • *Salmonella* • SIV – swine influenza • African swine fever • Classical swine fever
Breathing more per minute	• APP – *Actinobacillus pleuropneumoniae* • Heat stress • PMWS
Bush foot	• Bush foot

Continued ▸

MAIN CLINICAL SIGN	Causative disorders/agents
Coughing	• *Actinobacillus suis* • APP – *Actinobacillus pleuropneumoniae* • Gastric ulcer • *Mycoplasma hyopneumoniae* – enzootic pneumonia – PRDC • Porcine respiratory coronavirus • Pseudorabies – Aujeszky's disease • Swine influenza – SIV
Deviation	• Acquired deviation • Progressive atrophic rhinitis
Diarrhoea	• Coccidiosis • Colitis • Dysentery • *Escherichia coli* • Ileitis – PIA • PED • Rotavirus • *Salmonella* • TGE/PED
Diarrhoea-yellow	• Coccidiosis • *Escherichia coli* • *Salmonella*
Diarrhoea-red blood	• Clostridia enteritis • Swine dysentery
Diarrhoea-black	• Ileitis – PIA • Ulcer
Diarrhoea-clear	• Rotavirus • TGE/PED
Diarrhoea-gray	• Colitis • *Escherichia coli* • Ileitis – PIA
Discharge-nasal	• *Actinobacillus pleuropneumoniae* – blood • Foot and mouth disease • Progressive atrophic rhinitis – blood • SIV – Swine influenza
Discharge-anal	• See causes of diarrhoea
Discharge-aural	• Mange

Continued ▸

MAIN CLINICAL SIGN	Causative disorders/agents
Discharge-mouth	• *Actinobacillus pleuropneumoniae* – blood • Foot and mouth disease
Discharge-ocular	• Bowel oedema • Progressive atrophic rhinitis • SIV – Swine influenza
Discharge-vulva	• Brucellosis • Cystitis • Vulval discharges
Granuloma	• Granuloma
Greasy skin	• Greasy pig disease
Haematoma	• Aural haematoma
Lame high up	• Glässer's • Lame sows • *Mycoplasma* arthritis
Lame low down	• Erysipelas • Foot and mouth disease • Glässer's • Lame sows
Limb shape	• Conformation
Loose faeces	• Colitis • Ileitis – PIA • *Salmonella*
Lymph nodes swollen	• Lymphosarcoma • PMWS • PRRSv
Mastitis	• *Actinobacillus suis* • *Escherichia coli* • Streptococci species
Meningitis	• Glässer's • *Streptococcus* meningitis
Mucus	• Colitis • Dysentery • Ileitis – PIA
Mummified	• Parvovirus • PRRSv

Continued ▸

MAIN CLINICAL SIGN	Causative disorders/agents
Neurological problems	• Congenital tremor • Middle ear disease • Pseudorabies – Aujeszky's disease • Stroke
Noise change	• Bowel oedema • *Streptococcus* meningitis
Oedema swellings	• Bowel oedema • Glässer's
Orchitis	• Brucellosis
Paraplegia	• Sow paraplegia • Splay legs
Parasites seen	• *Ascaris suum* • Lice
Pig grouping (pigs lying in a pile)	• Salt poisoning – water deficiency
Refusal of feed	• Almost all conditions
Scratching	• Allergy • Lice • Mange
Skin bluing	• *Actinobacillus suis* • APP – *Actinobacillus pleuropneumoniae* • Erysipelas • Glässer's • *Salmonella* • *Streptococcus* infections
Skin colour change	• Gastric ulcer • Ileitis • Leptospirosis
Skin erosions	• Leg injuries
Skin necrosis	• Glässer's • *Streptococci*
Skin patches	• Erysipelas • PDNS • Pityriasis rosea • Ringworm • African swine fever • Classical swine fever

Continued ▸

MAIN CLINICAL SIGN	Causative disorders/agents
Skin scaly	• Essential oil deficient • Lice • Mange
Sneezing	• *Pasteurella* • Progressive atrophic rhinitis • Swine influenza
Stillborn	• *Parvovirus* • PRRSv
Sudden death	• APP – *Actinobacillus pleuropneumoniae* • Clostridial enteritis • Dysentery • Erysipelas • Glässer's • Mulberry heart • *Pasteurella/Streptococci* pneumonia • Pseudorabies – Aujeszky's disease • African swine fever • Classical swine fever
Swollen abdomen	• Glässer's • Rectal stricture • Salmonella • Twist
Swollen joints	• Erysipelas • Glässer's • *Mycoplasma* arthritis • Streptococci infections
Tumour	• Tumours
Urine-blood	• Pyelonephritis
Urine-smokey	• Cystitis
Vesicles and blisters	• Foot and mouth disease
Vomiting	• Gastric ulcer • *Salmonella* • TGE/PED
Vulva-necrotic	• Mycotoxins
Vulva-swollen	• Mycotoxins

Health alarm list

The vet should be notified as soon as possible if any of the following signs are seen by a member of the unit staff and verified by the manager.

> This aims to reduce any time delay between an outbreak and effective treatment.

Any age group

The development of lameness in pens or groups of pigs.

Blisters on the snout or excessive salivation in pens or groups of pigs.

Sows

Four or more sows off their feed with an elevated temperature.

Four or more sows breathing rapidly and with obvious respiratory distress.

Four or more sows aborting within seven days.

Suckling herd

A noticeable rise in pre-weaning mortality over a two week period.

Growing-finishing herd

A noticeable rise in post-weaning mortality over a two week period.

Scour spreading through any age of pigs, particularly if containing blood.

A marked rise in the number and severity of pigs coughing or with laboured breathing.

Three or more unexpected deaths in one day.

The numbers chosen are for a 10 sow a week batch farm (250 sows).

Compromised pig decision tree

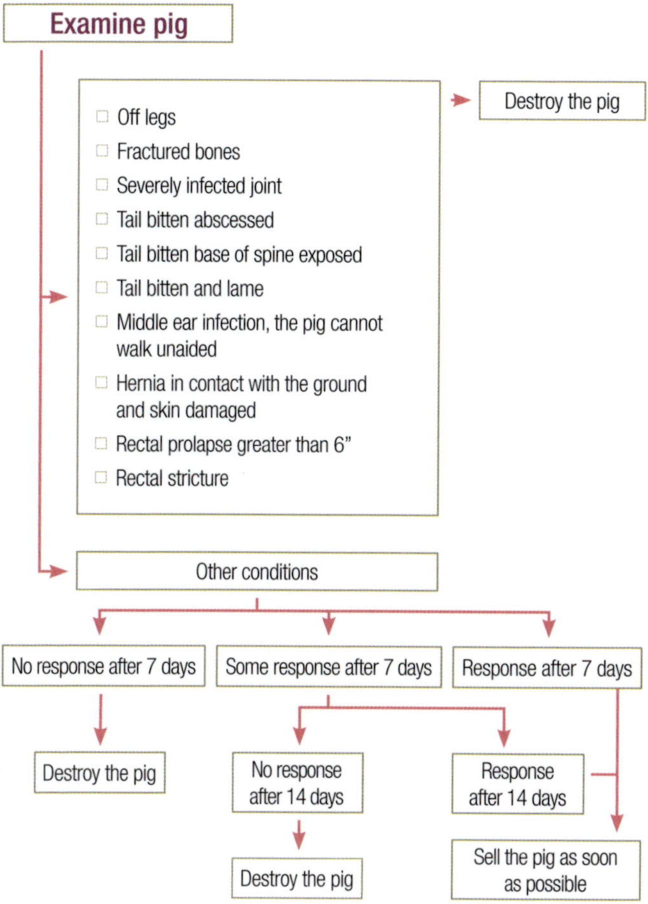

Euthanasia methods

Age	Piglet (less than 3 weeks)	Weaner (less than 10 weeks)	Grower (less than 75 kg)	Finisher	Adult
Blunt trauma	Acceptable	Unacceptable	Unacceptable	Unacceptable	Unacceptable
Carbon dioxide	Acceptable	Acceptable	Unacceptable	Unacceptable	Unacceptable
Gunshot	Unacceptable	Acceptable	Acceptable	Acceptable	Acceptable
Captive bolt	Unacceptable	Unacceptable	Acceptable	Acceptable	Acceptable
Anaesthetic	Acceptable	Acceptable	Acceptable	Acceptable	Acceptable

* Check against the legislation applicable in each country.

- Acceptable methods.
- Unacceptable methods.

Note pigs euthanised with a captive bolt should be exsanguinated, a captive bolt only stuns.
Anaesthetic euthanasia is only available under the supervision of a veterinarian.

Major disorders of the pig by age/group

The table indicates where the disorder is most likely to be seen. In naïve herds any animal age group can show clinical signs of a new disease.

It is always important to consult with your veterinarian if you suspect any signs of disease.

Pathogen	P	W	G/F	A
Actinobacillus pleuropneumoniae	Relatively rare	Uncommon	Relatively common	Relatively rare
Actinobacillus suis	Relatively common	Relatively common	Relatively rare	Relatively rare
Actinobaculum suis	Relatively rare	Relatively rare	Relatively rare	Relatively common
African swine fever	Relatively common	Relatively common	Relatively common	Relatively common
Ascaris suum	Uncommon	Uncommon	Relatively common	Relatively rare
Aujeszky's disease (pseudorabies)	Relatively rare	Relatively common	Relatively common	Uncommon
Bordetella bronchiseptica	Relatively rare	Relatively common	Relatively rare	Relatively rare
Borrelia spiralis	Relatively rare	Relatively rare	Uncommon	Relatively common
Brachyspira hyodysenteriae	Relatively rare	Uncommon	Relatively common	Relatively rare
Brachyspira pilosicoli	Relatively rare	Uncommon	Relatively common	Relatively rare
Classical swine fever (hog cholera)	Relatively common	Relatively common	Relatively common	Relatively common
Clostridium difficile	Relatively common	Relatively rare	Relatively rare	Relatively rare
Clostridium perfringens	Relatively common	Relatively rare	Relatively rare	Relatively rare
Congenital tremor virus?	Relatively common	Relatively rare	Relatively rare	Relatively rare
Cytomegalovirus	Relatively common	Relatively rare	Relatively rare	Relatively rare
Escherichia coli F18 Ste2x (bowel oedema)	Relatively rare	Relatively common	Relatively rare	Relatively rare
E. coli (cystitis)	Relatively rare	Relatively rare	Relatively rare	Relatively common
E. coli (diarrhoea)	Relatively common	Relatively common	Relatively rare	Relatively rare
Epidemic diarrhoea virus	Relatively common	Relatively common	Relatively common	Relatively common
Erysipelothrix rhusiopathiae	Relatively rare	Uncommon	Relatively common	Relatively common
Foot and mouth virus	Relatively common	Relatively common	Relatively common	Relatively common
Haematopinus suis	Relatively common	Relatively common	Relatively common	Relatively common
Haemophilus parasuis	Relatively rare	Relatively common	Uncommon	Relatively rare
Hyostrongylus rubidis	Relatively rare	Relatively rare	Relatively rare	Relatively common
Isospora suis	Relatively common	Uncommon	Relatively rare	Relatively rare
Lawsonia intracellularis	Relatively rare	Uncommon	Relatively common	Relatively rare
Leptospirosis	Relatively rare	Uncommon	Uncommon	Uncommon
Metastrongylus apri	Relatively rare	Relatively rare	Relatively rare	Relatively common
Mycoplasma hyopneumoniae	Relatively rare	Relatively rare	Relatively common	Relatively rare

Continued ▸

P = piglet W = weaner G/F = grow/finish A = adult pig

Relatively common Uncommon Relatively rare

Pathogen	P	W	G/F	A
Mycoplasma hyosynoviae	Relatively rare	Relatively rare	Uncommon	Relatively rare
Mycoplasma suis	Relatively rare	Uncommon	Uncommon	Uncommon
Oesophagostomum dentatum	Relatively rare	Relatively rare	Relatively rare	Relatively common
Parvovirus	Relatively rare	Relatively rare	Relatively rare	Relatively common
Pasteurella multocida (toxigenic) (PAR)	Relatively rare	Relatively common	Relatively rare	Relatively rare
Pasteurellosis	Relatively rare	Uncommon	Relatively common	Relatively rare
PMWS	Relatively rare	Relatively common	Uncommon	Relatively rare
Porcine circovirus 1 and 2	Relatively common	Relatively common	Relatively common	Relatively common
PRRSv	Relatively common	Relatively common	Relatively common	Relatively common
Ringworm	Relatively rare	Relatively rare	Uncommon	Relatively common
Rotavirus	Relatively common	Relatively rare	Relatively rare	Relatively rare
Salmonellosis	Relatively rare	Uncommon	Relatively common	Uncommon
Sarcoptes scabiei	Relatively rare	Uncommon	Relatively common	Relatively common
Spirochaetal colitis	Relatively rare	Uncommon	Relatively common	Relatively rare
Staphylococcus hyicus	Relatively rare	Relatively common	Relatively rare	Relatively rare
Stephanurus dentatum	Uncommon	Uncommon	Uncommon	Uncommon
Streptococcus (abscess)	Relatively common	Relatively common	Relatively common	Relatively common
Streptococcus (arthritis)	Relatively common	Uncommon	Relatively rare	Relatively rare
Streptococcus suis (joint ill)	Relatively common	Relatively rare	Relatively rare	Relatively rare
Streptococcus suis (meningitis)	Uncommon	Relatively common	Uncommon	Relatively rare
Strongyloides ransomi	Uncommon	Relatively common	Uncommon	Relatively rare
Swine influenza virus	Relatively rare	Relatively rare	Relatively common	Relatively common
Swine pox virus	Relatively rare	Relatively common	Uncommon	Relatively rare
Teschovirus	Relatively rare	Relatively rare	Relatively rare	Uncommon
TGE Transmissible gastroenteritis	Relatively common	Relatively common	Uncommon	Uncommon
Toxoplasma gondii	Uncommon	Uncommon	Uncommon	Uncommon
Trichinella spiralis	Relatively rare	Uncommon	Uncommon	Uncommon
Trichuris suis	Relatively rare	Relatively common	Relatively common	Relatively rare
Trueperella pyogenes	Relatively common	Relatively common	Relatively common	Relatively common

P = piglet W = weaner G/F = grow/finish A = adult pig

Relatively common Uncommon Relatively rare

Farrowing area checklist

There are 3 key questions regarding farrowing management:

	Question	Correct answer	Problem
1	What is the level of scour in piglets?	None	Draughts, chilling, colostrum management
2	How much food is eaten on day 18 by the sow?	> 10 kg per day	Water availability, feeding policies – lactation and gestation and temperature management
3	Number and weight of weaned piglets per batch?	> 12 per place 90 kg (27 days)	Pig flow, diseases issues in lactation, lactation feed intake, breeding management

Checklist for the farrowing area-indoors

Biosecurity	• All-in/all-out procedures • Use of footbaths • Building maintenance
Stock	• Empty farrowing places? • Sows' body condition at entry • Sow condition at weaning • Are any sows not in pig? • Late or early farrowings • Udder oedema, mastitis or metritis • Quality of piglets at birth • Sow mortality, prolapse, etc. • Sow health problems • Litter sizes, still-births, mummified piglets • Congenital conditions • Scour levels. Treatments. • Health of piglets, evenness of growth • Respiratory disease, rhinitis, pneumonia • Parasites, fly control • Numbers weaned • Weaning weight

Continued ▸

Water	• Water availability
Food	• Feeding protocols • Feeder management – mouldy feed • Overfed sows
Floor	• Dry floors • General hygiene
Air	• Room temperature • Cooling systems • Creep/heat mat temperatures • Evidence of draughts
Stockman-ship	• Farrowing problems • Are other procedures being done properly? • Are medication procedures being carried out properly e.g. mange, worming, vaccination?
Others	....

A checklist for the farrowing area – outdoors

Biosecurity	• Paddock management
Stock	• Accuracy of recording
Sows	• Behavioural problems • Body condition, body score • Born alive, dead, reared • Efficiency of breeding female • Gilt mothering qualities • Lactation ration used • Management efficiency • Mastitis, agalactia • Treatment required • Variability of body condition

Continued ▸

Piglets	• Born dead • Effects of bedding on viability • Losses due to foxes, crows • Iron injections • Management at farrowing • Mortality (%) • Quality of piglets at weaning • Savaging • Scour • Stolen piglets • Treatments required • Numbers weaned • Weight weaned
Water	• Depth of water in trough • Adequate water provisions
Food	• Food clean and adequately provided • Food distribution adequate to prevent fighting
Floor	• Bedding type quality amount-dryness • Level ground • Nose ring to prevent digging • Provision of solid floors • Size of the huts or arks for breed of sow • Soil type/nesting
Air	• Air flow, draughts, condensation • Wallows/shade • Sitting against prevailing wind • Insulation • Door flaps • Fenders
Stockman-ship	• Farrowing problems? • Processing procedures done properly?

Nursery checklist

	Question	Correct answer	Causes of variation
1	Are lying patterns normal?	Where expected	Presence of draughts
2	What is the growth rate in 1st week post-weaning?	Feed intake 300 g/day	Stockmanship inadequate
3	Is any evidence of vice?	Absence	Stress management
4	Mortality (%)?	Below 3 %	Presence of disease
5	Weight at 10 weeks of age?	30 kg	Feed intake and stress management

Checklist for the nursery inside

Biosecurity	• All-in/all-out practiced • Vermin control • Fly control
Stock	• Age and weight at weaning • Evenness of growth • Growth of the pig in the first ten days post-weaning • Respiratory diseases, rhinitis, pneumonia • Enteric diseases • Condition of the faeces • Skin conditions, mange, greasy pig disease • Lameness
Water	• Water availability
Feed	• Feed, access, type and quality
Floor	• Stocking density
Air	• Lying patterns of the pigs • Defecation patterns • Environmental temperature • Temperature variation with growth • Insulation • Lighting patterns
Stockmanship	• Welfare aspects
Others	....

Grow/finish checklist

	Question	Correct answer	Causes of variation
1	Weight adequate for age	Yes	Growth patterns
2	Evenness of batch	Yes	Growth patterns
3	Hospital pen management	Correct	Welfare
4	Evidence of vices	No	Draughts, environment problems

Checklist for the growing and finishing areas – indoors

Biosecurity	• All-in/all-out practiced
Stock	• Assess weight for age • Evenness of growth • Nutrition and growth in different houses • Appearance of the pigs skin-mange, hair growth • Appearance of faeces • Respiratory diseases • Enteric diseases • Diseases, mortality, prolapse • Vices present • Culls • Parasites
Water	• Provision of water
Food	• Application of feed and types • Evidence of over-feeding • Food wasted? • Feed conversion efficiency
Floor	• Stocking density • Daily liveweight gain
Air	• Lying patterns of the pigs • Temperature fluctuations • Evidence of draughts
Stockmanship	• Effect of movement of pigs • Hospital provisions
Slaughter	• Roadway good • Transport system in use • Number of pigs sold • Deadweight achieved
Others	....

Checklist for the dry/gestating sow area

	Question	Correct answer	Causes of variation
1	Vulvar discharges 14-21 days post-service	< 5 %	Reproductive performance
2	Number of lame sows	< 2 %	Condition of floors
3	Crates too small for the sows	No	Stress management

Checklist for the dry/gestation sow area – indoors

Biosecurity	• Gilt and boar introduction
Stock	• Assess the environment – temperatures, humidity • Housing problems, • Welfare problems • General sow contentment or restlessness • Chronic mastitis • Vulval discharges • Sows not in pig • Sows repeating • Abortions • Oestrus abnormalities • Condition of the faeces • Culls. Reasons for and causes • Mortality levels and causes • Prolapse
Water	• Water provision adequate
Feed	• Body condition, feed levels, inappetance
Floor	• Evidence of broken floors
Air	• Temperature of the gestation area
Stockmanship	• Vaccination programmes • Hospital area provisions
Others	....

Diseases of pigs notifiable to the OIE

- ☐ African swine fever
- ☐ Anthrax (*Bacillus anthracis*)
- ☐ Aujeszky's disease/Pseudorabies
- ☐ Brucellosis (*Brucella suis*)
- ☐ Classical swine fever
- ☐ Echinococcosis/hydatidosis (*Echinococcus granulosus*)
- ☐ Foot and mouth disease
- ☐ Japanese B encephalitis
- ☐ New world screwworm (*Cochliomyia hominivorax*)
- ☐ Nipah virus encephalitis
- ☐ Old world screwworm (*Chrysomya bezziana*)
- ☐ Paratuberculosis
- ☐ Porcine cysticercosis (*Taenia solium*)
- ☐ Porcine reproductive and respiratory syndrome
- ☐ Q fever
- ☐ Rabies
- ☐ Rinderpest
- ☐ Swine vesicular disease
- ☐ Transmissible gastroenteritis
- ☐ Trichinellosis (*Trichinella spiralis*)
- ☐ Vesicular stomatitis

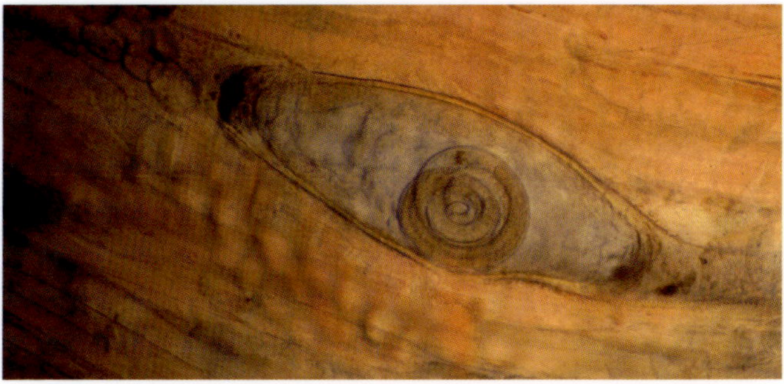

Zoonotic diseases of pigs

- ☐ Anthrax
- ☐ Brucellosis
- ☐ *Camplyobacter jejuni*
- ☐ Chagas' disease (*Trypanosoma cruzi*)
- ☐ *Chlamydia*
- ☐ *Clostridium difficile*
- ☐ *Clostridium perfringens* type A
- ☐ Ebola (Reston)
- ☐ Erysipelas
- ☐ *Escherichia coli*
- ☐ Japanese B encephalitis
- ☐ Louping ill
- ☐ Leptospirosis
- ☐ Melioidosis (*Burkholderia pseudomallei*)
- ☐ Nipah disease
- ☐ Pasteurellosis
- ☐ Rabies
- ☐ Ringworm
- ☐ Salmonellosis
- ☐ *Streptococcus suis*
- ☐ Swine influenza
- ☐ Trypanosomiasis
- ☐ *Taenia solium*
- ☐ Toxoplasmosis
- ☐ *Trichinella spiralis*
- ☐ Tuberculosis
- ☐ Vesicular diseases

Suspected exotic disease protocols

Client suspects an unusual or potentially exotic disease

- ☐ Request client seal the property.
- ☐ Place keep out notices at all public entrances.
- ☐ Request that all personnel remain at the property until the vet arrives.

Veterinarians' responsibility

- ☐ Wear disposable outer clothing and only wear farm boots.
- ☐ Take a suitable disinfectant concentrate in the car.
- ☐ Ensure you have a camera (which can be washed) and mobile phone which works.
- ☐ Ensure you have a rectal thermometer.
- ☐ Upon arrival examine stock carefully.
- ☐ Photograph and catalogue any observed clinical signs.

Veterinarian suspects an unusual or exotic disease

- ☐ Phone practice to inform partners. Email photographs of clinical signs.
- ☐ Phone Government Agriculture Veterinarian (get the local number and put on your phone).
- ☐ Provide full name and address of the farm and GSP location if possible.
- ☐ Provide clear details of how to get to the location of animals and farm.
- ☐ Email photographs and clinical details of the observed lesions.

Before the arrival of the Department of Agriculture Veterinarian (unless otherwise authorised)

- ☐ Stop movement of all animals from and to the farm.
- ☐ Stop all movement of vehicles from the farm.

- ☐ Divert all movement of all vehicles that are to arrive at the farm – such as feed trucks, milk tanker, etc.
- ☐ Ensure farm perimeter entry points prohibit vehicle movements – for example place tractor across entrance, ensure signs are in place, if necessary place stockpeople at entrance.
- ☐ Proceed with a detailed clinical examination of all the other stock on the farm – all species.

Leaving the farm

- ☐ Follow all advice given by the Government Agriculture Veterinarian.
- ☐ Leave disposable overalls.
- ☐ Leave farm boots.
- ☐ Leave rectal thermometer.
- ☐ Do not remove any items contaminated with faeces or blood.
- ☐ If necessary, rewrite notes on clean paper.
- ☐ Provide counselling and support to the client with regard to possibility that the suspect disease is confirmed.
- ☐ Implement suitable additional biosecurity measures.
- ☐ Spray car wheels and wheel hubs with a suitable disinfectant.
- ☐ On the way home wash car in hot steam car wash.
- ☐ Double wash all clothing with detergent.
- ☐ Shower thoroughly – minimum 3 minutes – note watch and glasses.
- ☐ Thoroughly clean and disinfect all equipment removed from the farm.

During routine visit the veterinarian suspects an exotic or unusual animal disease

- ☐ Proceed as indicated in the part Veterinarians' responsibilty (items 3 to 6).
- ☐ Do not take personal boots and overalls from the farm.
- ☐ Ensure you have a small supply of a suitable disinfectant in the car at all times.

3 General ideas

Gilt litters vs. sow litters

The offspring of gilts and sows do not have the same prospects in life.

Expectation of offspring	Gilt	Sow
Litter weight (kg)	96	100
Finishing rate (%)	91	96
Days to 115 kg	162	154
Growth rate (g/day)	670	700
FCR	2.7	2.4

Gilt piglets are more likely to succumb to pathogens and diseases.

It is important that when an outbreak of disease, such as pneumonia, occurs in a batch of finishing pigs check what was the component of gilt in the batch. A critical percentage occurs when a batch has 30 % or more gilts.

To stabilise the finishing herd it is vital to standardise the gilt percentage per batch.

If the farm has a PRRSv outbreak, ensure all gilt litters also receive colostrum from adjacent sows.

In PRRSv positive farms gilts must not be excreting the virus when they enter the breeding herd.

Split suckling

Colostrum intake is vital to survival of pigs. Each piglet needs a minimum of at least 100 ml of colostrum. Blood IgG concentration should be > 10 mg/ml.

A system needs to be used to ensure that all the pigs get adequate colostrum.

Ensure that the farrowing house is well prepared for the forthcoming farrowing.

The heat mats or creep lights need to be placed both behind the sow and the creep area already dry and warm at 30 °C. Adequate ambient room temperature for the sows is around 20 °C.

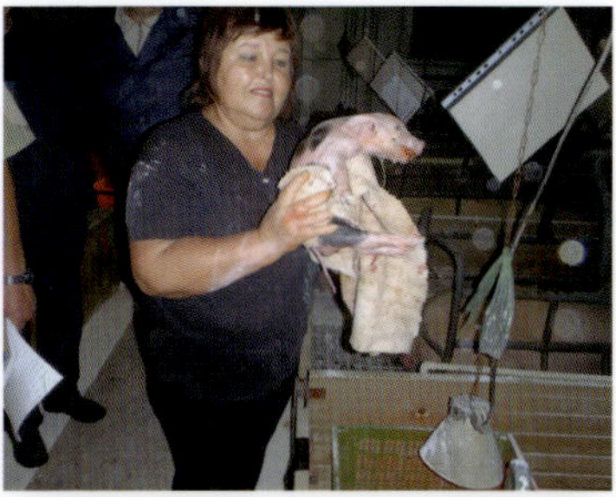

Be there at parturition; collect and dry piglets as they are being born.

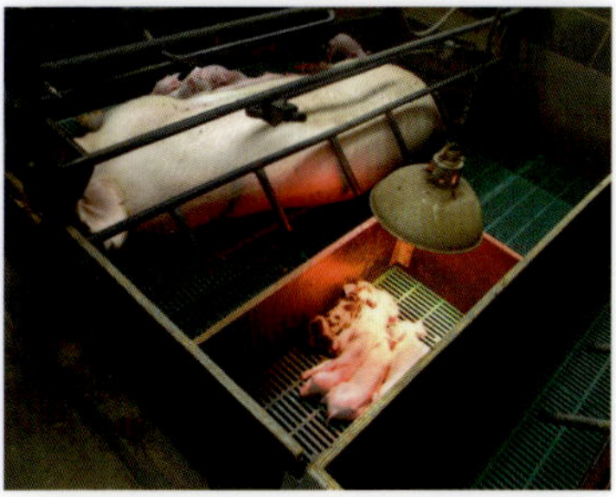

Place them into a basket under a heat lamp with the ambient air in the basket at 30-35 °C.

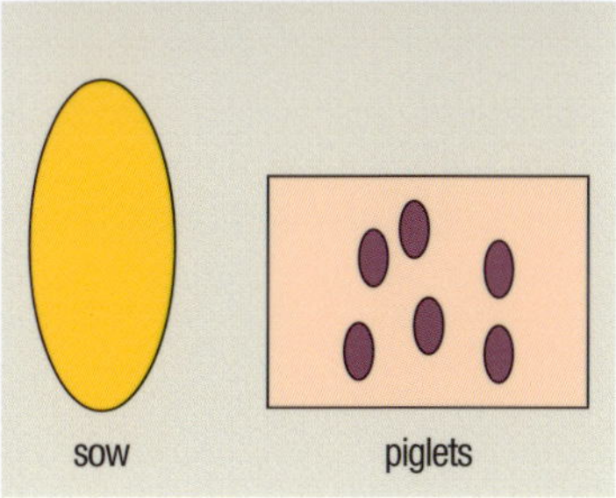

Collect all the pigs born over the first two hours, dry and place in a basket under a heat lamp.

After 2 hours, mark the pigs and release the warm and dried pigs onto the sow to suckle (group 1). Collect all the newly born piglets, dry and place into the basket under a heat lamp (group 2).

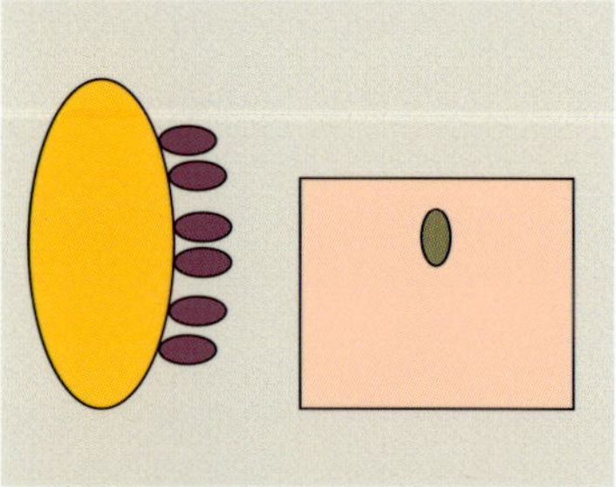

After 2 hours collect all the pigs which have been suckling. Release the second batch of pigs onto the sow to suckle. Place group 1 pigs into the warming basket.

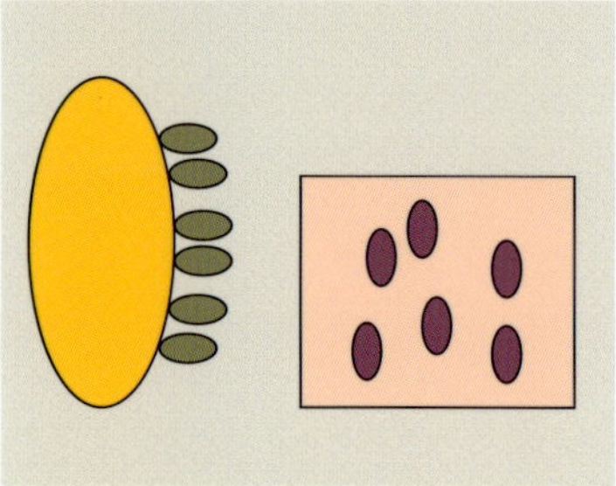

As new piglets are born continue to dry and place in warming basket – group 3 pigs. Mark with a different colour to group 1 pigs.

By 4 hours normally farrowing should have been completed.

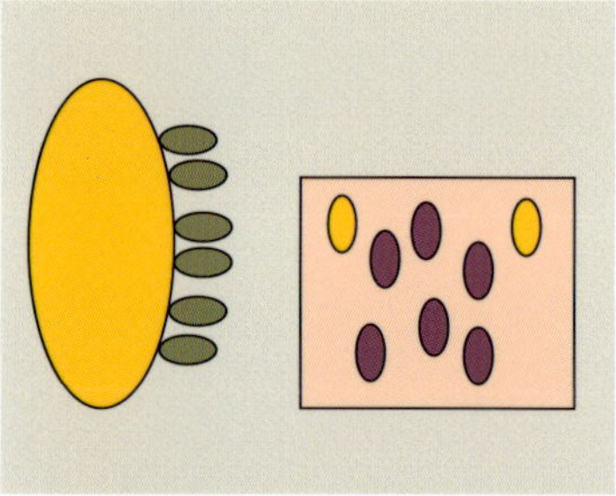

Collect group 2 pigs and place in warming basket.

Release group 3 pigs (if any) onto the sow to suckle for 30 minutes. Ensure all piglets suckle.

If there is no group 3 pigs or only a couple apply commonsense to suckling behaviour.

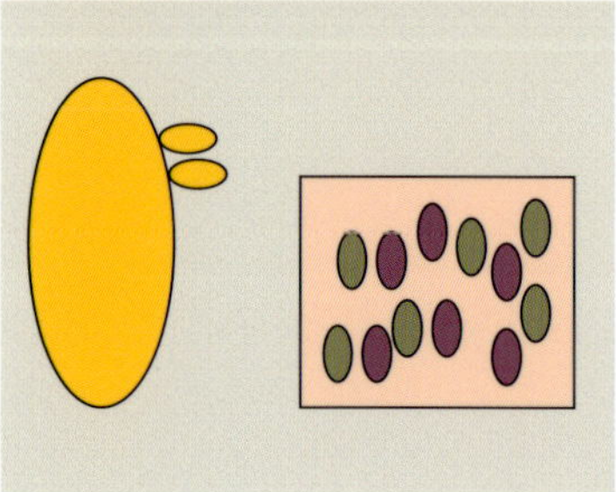

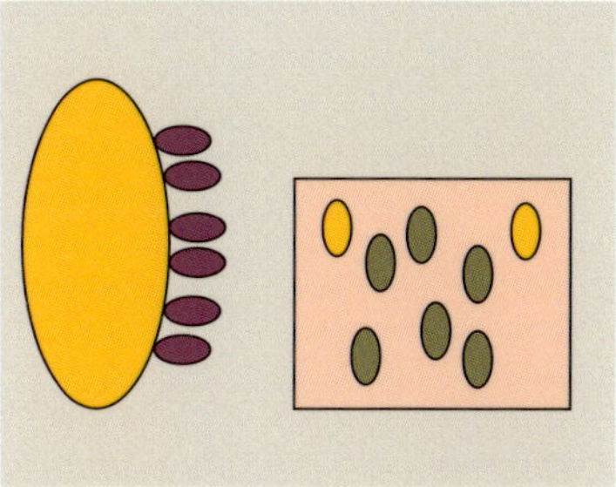

Release group 1 piglets onto the sow for 30 minutes. Ensure all piglets have drunk colostrum.
Collect and place in warming basket. Release group 2 and group 3 piglets onto the sow for 30 minutes. Ensure all piglets have drunk colostrum.

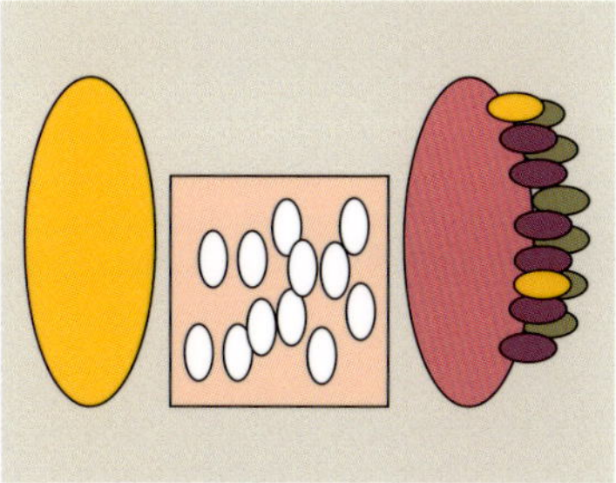

1st parity litter: collect a mature sow's litter and place into a warming basket. Place the entire gilts litter (group 1, 2 and 3) onto the sow to suckle for 1 hour.

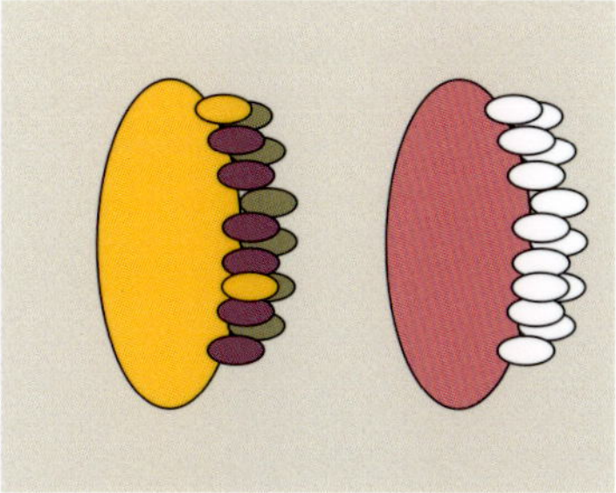

Collect the parity 1 piglets and return to original mother. Release sows litter back onto their original mother.

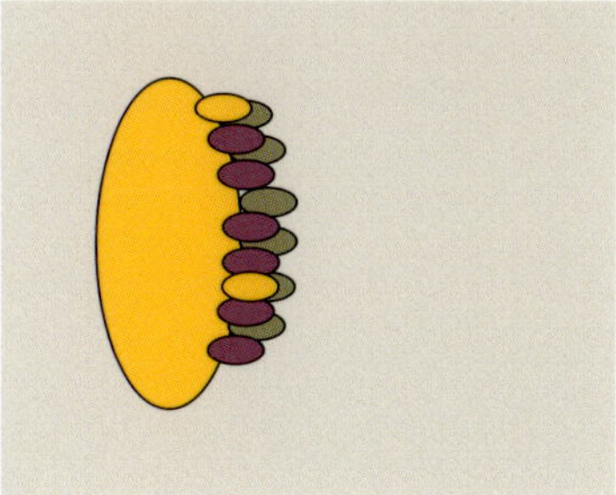

Sow litter: after the 5 hours of split suckling, allow all piglets free access to the sow.

Fostering and sorting can be completed after 18 to 24 hours.

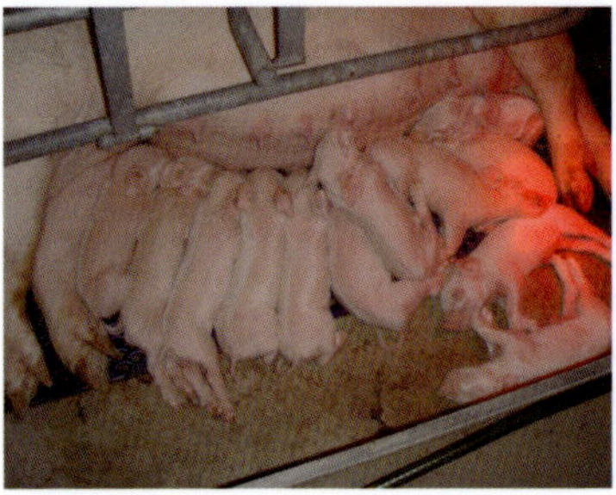

The gut closure of the antibodies and maternal cells occurs 6-12 hours after the first suckle – not from the moment of birth.

The provision of sow colostrum to gilt piglets reduces their mortality in the finishing unit and increased their growth rates.

Forward fostering routines

Within 24 hours of birth

- Even litter sizes between sows and gilts which have finished farrowing 24 hours previously.
- Only provide piglets to correspond to teat numbers and numbers normally reared by parity.
- Administer warm colostrum to each piglet to be fostered.
- Ensure all gilts have 12 piglets each for the first week at least.

On the day of weaning

1. Wean this week's pigs (say 27 day old piglets).
2. From the next weeks pigs to wean (say 18 day old piglets), select and wean the strongest litter, ensuring there are 12 pigs on the litter and that all the sow's teats work. Ensure the sow's temperament is suitable for fostering. This is sow 1.

3 Select one litter of strong piglets from a sow with about 11 day old piglets. This is sow 2.

4 Ensure all additional piglets are ear notched.

5 Move these piglets forward onto sow 1.

6 Encourage the sow to suckle the 11 day old piglets by rubbing her teat line, observing and talking to the sow.

7 From piglets of around 7 days select and wean the strongest litter, ensuring there are 11 pigs on the litter and that all her teats work. Ensure the sow's temperament is suitable for fostering. This is sow 3.

8 Ensure all additional piglets are ear notched and those less than 7 days of age are teeth clipped.

9 Move these piglets forward onto sow 2.

10 Encourage the sow to suckle the 7 day old piglets by rubbing her teat line, observing and talking to the sow.

11 Administer warm colostrum to each piglet.

12 Move the weakest ten 7 day old or less piglets from their mothers and foster onto sow 3.

13 Ensure all additional piglets are ear notched and those less than 7 days of age are teeth clipped.

14 Encourage the sow to suckle the 7 day old piglets by rubbing her teat line, observing and talking to the sow.

15 Administer warm colostrum to each piglet.

16 Record fostering to weaning mortality.

17 It is essential that fostering routines do not interfere with all-in/all-out farrowing house practices.

18 Fostering is more successful if whole litters are moved.

19 Fostering should not be backwards. Older piglets must not be fostered back with younger piglets.

20 If adult sows are unable to rear 11+ piglets, investigate why.

Nursing patterns and consequences

What attracts new born piglets?

- Vocalisation of sows.
- Dark areas.
- Afterbirth and birth fluids.
- Piglets will follow the sow's hair patterns towards the teats.

Suckling after birth

Piglets contact teat as quickly as 3 minutes, but average 15 minutes to contact the udder and 30 minutes to contact the teat.

Milk is continuously available for several hours. Little aggression exists as pigs sample teats.

Cyclic milk ejection, approximately hourly, results in more aggression.

Cyclic nursing and suckling (approximately once every hour)

Sow	Piglets
☐ Slow grunting	☐ Assemble at udder
☐ Increase grunt rate	☐ Nosing and teat location
☐ Rapid increase in grunt rate	☐ Slow suckling
☐ Milk flow (15 sec)	☐ Rapid suckling
☐ Grunting declines	☐ Slow suckling or nosing
☐ Sleep or change position	☐ Fall sleep

Consequences of cyclic suckling

Fan noise may interfere with nursing cycles.

Piglets which miss a nursing do not eat until next bout.

Nurse within a room to synchronise.

Nursing can be stimulated by sound or massage.

Post-suckling massage related to milk yield and gut hormones.

Teat order

Teat order is established within 3 days and, usually, persists over 90 %. It is however less stable in large litters.

About 10 % of piglets use more than 1 teat, although suckling from multiple teat is more common in small litters.

Note that unused teats regress.

> When sow turns over, so does the piglet teat order. The order is teat – specific.

Consequences of a teat order

Stable teat orders lead to more uniform growth. Relative weight gain within litters depends on competition for teat.

Evening out litters by weights (first 3 days) or selective teeth clipping may reduce problematic piglets.

Unused teats produce less milk in subsequent lactation.

Mixing after day 9 make more difficult to re-make teat order (this takes 1-2 days). In natural state a sow would introduce her piglets to other sow's piglets around day 10. After day 14 the group of piglets join the main group.

When a pig is fostered after 48 hours, total litter performance is reduced.

Fostering is about two events:

- Foster after day 3 if you want more even litters (total litter weight will be reduced).
- Do not foster after day 3 if you want to maximise total litter weight (litter may be variable).

Enhancing piglet weaning weights

Feeding the dry sow

Increase feeding from day 90 to improve piglet birth weights. An extra 200 g at birth is worth about 6 days to slaughter. Restricting the feed intake of dry sows will also help lactation intake.

Adequate set up of farrowing accommodation

The farrowing accommodation must be very clean. It is essential to reduce as much as possible the disease risk. The farrowing area must also be set up to provide heat and a drying environment to the new born piglet. The farrowing area must be draught free. A heat source should be placed behind the back of the sow. Batch the system and colour code each batch.

Colostrum intake

Adequate colostrum intake and colostrum quality is the key to giving the piglet a good start.

Prompt feed intake

40 % of pre-weaning mortality is associated with malnutrition.

Feeding the lactating sow

To ensure good growth rates in the piglets, adequate milk production is needed for each day of life. Aim for a consumption of around 11 kg by day 18 of lactation (gilts may only achieve 9 kg).

> Adhere to a lactation diet, use an agreed feeding curve and a known quality feed.

Check water supply regularly: milk is 80 % water. Piglets are 85 % water. Lysine and valine concentrations may have a direct influence on weaning weight (1.3 % lysine and 1.3 % valine are recommended).

Barley based diets may help sows milk better with less problems post-farrowing.

Hygiene

To have an adequate hygiene may reduce risk of disease.

Piglets have two major options with protein intake: lay down lean tissue or produce antibodies.

Hygiene is not just about the initial set up, it is also cleaning while the piglets are in the room, i.e. prompt removal of scour. Having different brushes and scrapes for each room is a good option. Batch production and having a colour code for each batch, including equipment, are good routines as well.

Creep feeding

Creep feed 3 times a day with a good quality creep. Start this feeding from day 14, with little quantities served regularly. Use a creep tray (which is sterilised between batches and litters). Creep feeding has to be kept cool.

Proposed growth curve

Normal pig growth 180-250 g/day, but experimentally can be up to 500 g/day.

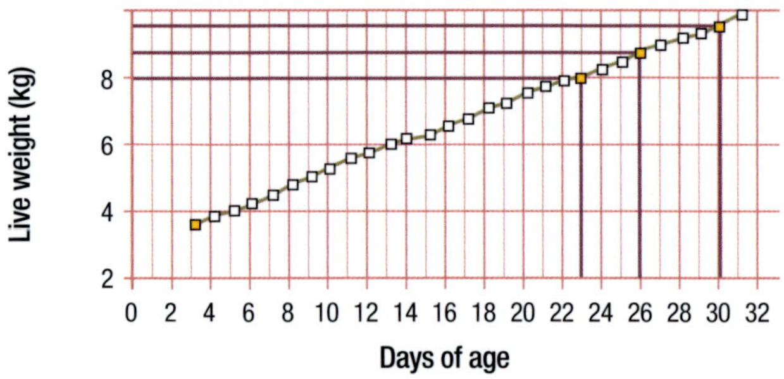

Water intake

Water intake is absolutely vital to weaning weights.

With sows fed a constant intake of feed and offered different amounts of water daily:

- 8 litres per day: piglet growth of 50 g/day.
- 16 litres per day: piglet growth of 200 g/day.
- 24 litres per day: piglet growth of 300 g/day.

All-in/all-out

This is the only way to attempt to achieve a reasonable standard of hygiene. You cannot pressure-wash while sows and piglets are in the room. Remember that moving piglets is moving disease.

Breeding programme

Change to a batch breeding programme rather than breeding by "opportunity". Only serve sufficient sows to fill the farrowing house as required. Divide farrowing area into usable blocks/batches, i.e. 24-day weaning gives a 5-week turn around.

Note that 5 week-batches with 4-week weaning or 4-week batches with 3-week weaning only require one farrowing room, thus all the batch farrowing places can be used at one time.

Cross-fostering

Very useful in the first 24 hours. After this time you must adhere to a pre-set protocol. Many cross-fostered piglets die and, as they spread pathogens, previously healthy piglets succumb.

Adequate identification of piglets is essential to ensure that cross-fostering is carried out effectively.

Ensure piglets are evenly shared between available sows. Ensure all gilts have 12 piglets for the first week.

Environment for piglets

Air: air temperature of 30 °C; air speed, zero.

Outdoors: check arc has no holes. Earth the sides of farrowing arcs to eliminate draughts.

No insulation increase LCT (Low Critical Temperature) 5 °C; wet floor increases LCT 10 °C; slow air movement (0,15 m/sec) increases LCT 6 °C.

Water: water- nipple 12 to 18 cm (4-6¨) from ground at 300 ml per min.

Feed: good quality creep, piglets have to be fed 3 times daily from day 14. Use a creep feeder. Store creep in the cool and dry off the ground.

Floor: insulated solid area is required. Ensure slatted area is not rough. Control flies indoors and foxes, seagulls and magpies outdoors. Fenders should fit well onto arc and ensure no piglet is able to escape.

Reduce disease

Good recognition of the disease causing a problem and prompt treatment are essential.

Willingness to submit live pigs for post-mortem investigations is needed.

Adequate feed-back and vaccine programmes.

Adequate medicine storage programmes.

Age of weaning

Is the post-weaning accommodation suitable for the weight of the pigs moving into the accommodation?

Time of day for feeding sows

Avoid feeding sow when ambient temperature is too hot, i.e. mid-day feeding as this will reduce total intake.

Gilt management

Provide the gilts with the stronger piglets.

Which day to wean?

Weaning day impact

The yellow boxes can be customised.
Dark pink boxes indicate weekends.
Grey boxes indicate ideal weekdays.

Day of weaning		Breeding		Farrowing		Weaning critical days	
Sunday	1	Thursday	Saturday	Sunday	Wednesday	Sunday	Wednesday
Monday	2	Friday	Sunday	Monday	Thursday	Monday	Thursday
Tuesday	3	Saturday	Monday	Tuesday	Friday	Tuesday	Friday
Wednesday	4	Sunday	Tuesday	Wednesday	Saturday	Wednesday	Saturday
Thursday	5	Monday	Wednesday	Thursday	Sunday	Thursday	Sunday
Friday	6	Tuesday	Thursday	Friday	Monday	Friday	Monday
Saturday	7	Wednesday	Friday	Saturday	Tuesday	Saturday	Tuesday

Wean-to-service interval	4	6	days
Gestation length	115	116	days
Weaning age	28		days
Critical period post-weaning	3		days

The farm should be orientated around maximising output.

Changing the farm to weaning on a Monday allows for maximum staff time to care and feed the newly weaned piglets. This can reduce finishing by 10 days.

Farrowing then occurs also during the middle of the week reducing the need to induce farrowing, which increases birth weights. However, breeding occurs over the weekend, but AI breeding routines can result in over 50 sows an hour being bred.

> Breeding is vital for the farm's success but not important from a time constraint view.

Tail biting and other vices

Here is a checklist of possible causes for tail biting.

- ☐ Check stocking density.
- ☐ Check tail length, in particular variability.
- ☐ Check feed particle size (target > 500 µm).
- ☐ Check salt (NaCl) concentration in feed. Levels of 0.9 % will result in problems; normal will be about 0.5 %.
- ☐ Check for evidence of a draught at pig heights (draught air speed > 0.2 m/sec).
- ☐ Check air quality (target - NH_3 < 20 ppm; H_2S < 10 ppm and CO_2 < 3,000 ppm).
- ☐ Check humidity (target between 50 and 75 %).
- ☐ Check light intensity.
- ☐ Check water supplies.
- ☐ Check feeder space availability.
- ☐ Check 24 hour temperature fluctuations.
- ☐ Mixing pigs.
- ☐ Moving pigs.

Scour pre-wean investigation

Area of concern

1 Note the timing of the scour – different pathogen agents affect the piglet on different days.

- ☐ 1 day after birth
- ☐ 3-7 days after birth
- ☐ > 10 days after birth

2 Note the type of scour and appearance of the anal ring.

- ☐ Blood
- ☐ Water
- ☐ Yellow/pasty
- ☐ Mucoid

3 Post-mortem examination of piglets. Acute piglets should be examined.

Environmental and management checks – the following may be associated with scouring piglets

- ☐ Almost any air movement is undesirable > 0.2 m/sec is a draught.
- ☐ Chilling of the piglets, check lying patterns and creep temperatures (ideally 30 °C).
- ☐ Variable temperatures in the creep.
- ☐ Damp floors particularly in the creep area.
- ☐ Poor colostrum intake.
- ☐ No milk in the sows, check udder line – mycotoxins and management.
- ☐ Degree of cross-fostering.
- ☐ Piglet treatments have not been clean enough, check cross-contamination between healthy and sick piglets.
- ☐ Infection transfer - is there a separate brush and scrape for each room/batch? Foot baths? Personal hygiene? Assign a colour code for each batch.

- Poor room cleaning between batches.
- Number of sows farrowing each batch, application of all-in/all-out and pig flow.
- Presence of udder oedema.
- Amount of navel bleeding.
- Type of iron injection utilised, lack of sufficient iron may encourage more post-weaning scour.
- Vaccine storage protocols.

The basic streaming concept

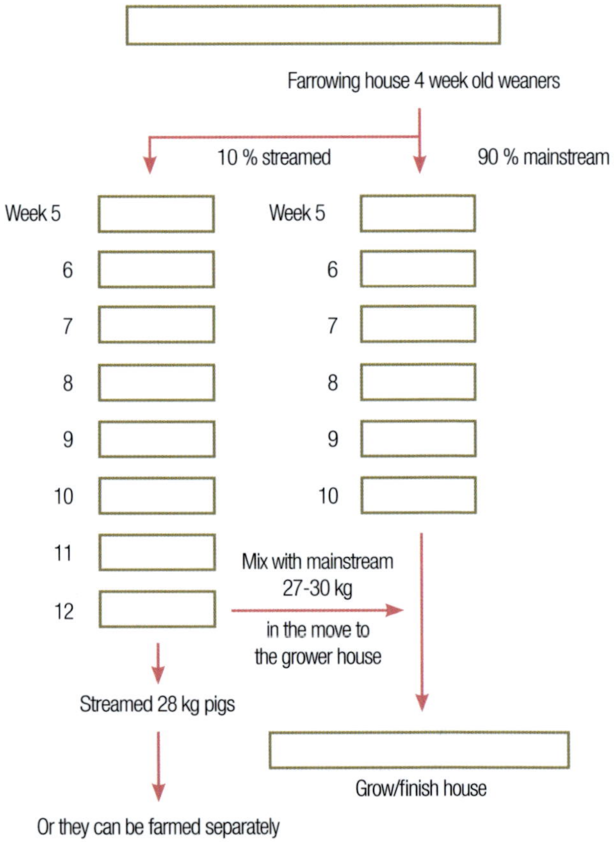

The two groups are in different buildings. This system allows the small pigs at weaning time to catch up with the normal pigs.

This is all-in/all-out by weight (but not by age).

> It is better to care for the small pigs post-weaning than resolving the problem in the finishing house.

The concept reduces the variation within a batch and can significantly reduce medication costs as generally only the smaller pigs require medication.

Scour post-weaning investigation

Area of concern

1. Note the timing of the diarrhoea. Many cases of diarrhoea actually start 5-7 days previously.
2. Note the type of diarrhoea and appearance of the anal ring:
   - ☐ Blood
   - ☐ Water
   - ☐ Yellow/pasty
   - ☐ Mucoid
   - ☐ Alkaline faeces: *Escherichia coli*
   - ☐ Acid faeces: viral
3. Post-mortem examination of weaners
   Euthanasia: acutely affected pigs should be examined, rather than looking only at chronically affected pigs with secondary problems.

Environmental and management checks

1 Post-weaning feeding routines.
Poor feed intake in the first week encourages gorging in the second week with protein overload of the gut (large bowel) and diarrhoea. Gruel feeding is essential combined with little and often feeding routines.

2 Hygiene of feeder – especially between batches.

3 Feeder space.
Inadequate feeder space increases aggression. Note behaviour in first 3 days.

4 Creep feeding and hygiene in the farrowing house.

5 Mycotoxins in feed and feed storage.
Note mycotoxins damage vitamins such as vitamin E and can affect the palatability of the feed.

6 Feed ingredients –zinc oxide presence, for example.

7 Is diarrhoea associated with a recent feed type change?

8 Water hygiene, especially between batches.

9 Almost any air movement is undesirable: > 0.2 m/sec is a draught in the sleeping area.

10 Chilling of the weaners: check lying patterns sleeping area temperatures (initially ideally > 27 °C) and defecation patterns.

11 Variable temperatures and high humidity in the sleeping area.

12 Damp floors/bedding particularly in the sleeping area.

13 Degree of cross-fostering pre-weaning.

14 Number of sows farrowing each week, application of all-in/all out and pig flow.

15 Age of piglets at weaning and the variability in age and weight.

16 Poor room cleaning between batches.

17 Infection transfer: is there a separate brush and scrape for each batch. Foot baths, personnel hygiene? Colour code batches.

18 Review vermin and fly control.

19 Equipment from weaner treatments that have not been clean enough. Check cross-contamination between healthy and sick pigs.

20 Type of iron injection utilised. Lack of sufficient iron may encourage more diarrhoea.

21 Medication issues. Vaccine storage protocols. Note maternal colostrum transfer post-weaning is poor for *E. coli* vaccines.

22 Review the presence of other pathogens, PRRSv and PCVAD/PMWS (Porcine circovirus associated diseases/Postweaning multisystemic wasting syndrome) for example.

23 Is a feed-back programme in place?

24 Check parity profile of the mother of weaners with diarrhoea.

Scour post-weaning treatment principles

Aims

Enhance pig's resistance to pathogens – or at least do nothing to reduce the pig's resistance.

Reduce pathogen load.

> Note most of the "pathogenic" organisms are "normal" in the environment.

Treatment and control protocols to reduce susceptible pigs

- ☐ Remove bottom 10 % smallest animals from the main group and house and manage differently.
- ☐ Review pig flow and ensure over and under-stocking is removed.
- ☐ Review weaner age and weights and enhance them.
- ☐ Review pre-weaning management to maximise health at weaning – review cross-fostering regimes in particular.
- ☐ Ensure iron administration pre-weaning adequate.
- ☐ Ensure all pigs are eating within 12 hours post-weaning.
- ☐ Ensure adequate feed space available – note newly weaned pigs eat as a group – automatic restrict feeding even if feed available "ad-lib".
- ☐ Ensure a warm, draught free sleeping area is available for all pigs.
- ☐ Provide warmer sleeping flooring – use of comfort boards, etc.

Enhance pig's resistance

- ☐ Presence of zinc oxide (ZnO) 2,500 g/t for first 2-3 weeks post-weaning.

> Note phytases may help reduce the ZnO required.

- ☐ Use acidifiers for the diet and water supplies.
- ☐ Use of probiotics (ensure they are alive) milk and yogurt products.
- ☐ Consider use of sterilise peat to act as an antitoxin/absorbent.
- ☐ Increase vitamin E concentration in feed to 250 ppm.
- ☐ Use suitable antimicrobial therapy.
- ☐ Ensure compliance with dose rate and treatment protocols. It may be necessary to treat whole groups of animals, including those that are not sick.
- ☐ Change genetics in cases of bowel oedema – *E. coli* F18.
- ☐ Consider vaccines against bowel oedema.

Miscellaneous

- □ If creep feeding is practiced pre-weaning: stop and review situation.
- □ Feed-back programmes using weaner faeces, including the diarrhoea, to gilts and sows 6 weeks pre-farrowing. Discuss this aspect with your veterinarian.
- □ If gilt litter's weaners are more prone to diarrhoea review management of these gilts – note particularly feed-back and immunity protocols.
- □ Review and possibly change creep/weaner feed type –meal, pellets, wet or dry size of pellets.

Reduce pathogen load

- □ Separate sick animals from main group as soon as possible to a hospital area.
- □ Provide electrolytes in water supply to sick pigs.
- □ Do not move sick pigs back into previous batch groups.
- □ Do not move recovered sick pigs back into main group until over 30 kg bodyweight.
- □ Practice rigid all-in/all-out.
- □ Adequate hygiene between batches – use of lime-washing.
- □ Ensure water lines are properly disinfected between batches.
- □ Ensure feeders are properly cleaned between batches.
- □ Ensure that there is no cross-contamination between batches through foot wear, brushes, scrapes or needles/syringes.
- □ Note hygiene of lying pads and sleeping boards.
- □ Enhance vermin and fly controls.
- □ Monitor weaners' rate and evenness of growth.

Meningitis – *Streptococcus suis* investigation

Undisturbed group of pigs	Examine and record lying pattern of undisturbed pigs – picture/video.
	Behaviour of pigs around the water supply – picture/video.
	Behaviour of pigs around the feeders – picture/video.
Stock	Clinical pigs respond to ceftiofur or penicillin.
Check for PRRSv	Blood results – note 21 days antibody delay.
PMWS/PCVAD	Ensure that the pigs were vaccinated at weaning – PCV2.
	Check vaccine purchases correspond to weaning numbers.
	Check medicine storage (2-8 °C).
Post-mortem	Ensure diagnosis correct – picture/video.
Sick pigs	Treatment of sick pigs.
	Movement of recovered pigs.
	Collect true mortality and morbidity figures.
Check weaning age and weight	Age at weaning.
	Weight at weaning.
Immunology	Feedback programme.
Pig flow	Collect true weaning/farrowing/breeding and gilt numbers by batch.
All-in/all-out	AIAO by pigs, water, feed, floor, air and medicine.
Medicines	Ensure needles and syringes not used between different groups/batches.
Water	Flow : 700 ml.
	Height: 13-30 cm (5-12 in).
	Number of drinkers.
	Cleaning programme between batches.
Floor	Nursery pigs need 0.3 m^2 per pig (to 30 kg).
	Cleaning programme between batches.

Continued ▸

Air	Temperature cooling curve 30 °C at entry. Cooling 1°C per week to 24 °C.
	Relative humidity (50-75 % RH).
	Gas heating – check colour of flame and CO concentration.
	Many farms with a meningitis problem staff have headaches.
	High dust and endotoxin issues.
	Note level of slurry under slats – how is the air flow from underneath slats?
	Draughts in the proposed sleeping areas.
	Examine defecation pattern of pigs.
	Smoke buildings and record air movement patterns-picture/video.
	Cleaning programme between batches.
Feed	Feed space (ad-lib 5 cm per pig of 30 kg and feeder management.
	What is the vitamin E concentration in the feed? Ideally 250 mg/kg.
	Gruel feeding regime 3-4 days post-weaning.
	Note feed space required immediately post-weaning – 10 cm (4 in) per pig as the pig initially feeds as a group and thus it is a restricted fed animal.
	Problem coincides with a change in diet/feed type and feed size.
	Cleaning programme between batches
Other problems	PRRSv, PCVAD/PMWS and mange are classical examples.
	Eliminate any additional stressors at weaning – weighing, tagging, bleeding.

Review "*The basic stockmanship guide: Pigs, Hogs and Swine*" (John Carr, Editorial Servet, 2013).

Enhancing post-weaning feed intake

It is essential to get the weaned pig rapidly adapted to its new existence post-weaning.

Feeding space – from weaning until day 3

Provide trough sufficient so that all the newly weaned pigs can eat at once. Provide 10 cm per pig – note the trough can allow pigs to eat from both sides – therefore 5 cm per pig. Thus for each 20 pigs provide 1 m of trough space.

The extra trough can be simply designed from plastic guttering; 12 cm wide supported by 35 cm long x 6 cm wide platforms.

If the floor is slotted, 15 cm long nails can be driven through the platform feet to hold the trough in place.

Components of the gruel

Solid

Any good quality early starter creep diet: 24 % protein, 18 DE. Highly digestible, ideally with a high milk component.

Liquid

Fresh water. It may be substituted with dairy by-products – out of date milk, cream, and yogurt for example. Chocolate by-products are also excellent.

	Consistency of the gruel		Volume of gruel per 100 pigs
	Water (%)	Solid (%)	
Day 1	80	20	2 litres every 2 hours
Day 2			2.5 litres every 2 hours
1-3 feed	50	50	
4-6 feed	40	60	
Day 3			2.5 litres every 3 hours
1-2 feed	30	70	
3-4 feed	20	80	
Day 4	0	100	2.5 kg of dry feed

From day 4: 100 % of water in troughs, to make pigs eat out of main feeders.

It is important to avoid contaminated water, which may cause feed refusal.

Feeding protocols

Day of weaning

1. Wean the pigs and allow 2 hours for the weaners to acclimatise to their new environment. Ideally make several drinkers leak so the weaners are attracted to them. No drinker should be elevated or requiring a step up. Turkey drinkers can be very useful.

2. After 2 hours go into the weaner pen and call the weaners by voice.

Tap on the feed bucket and pour the gruel into the trough, filling the whole length of the trough.

The weaners will rapidly come up to you and start swarming around you and the trough. Stay still and gently talk to the weaners.

It is essential that only sufficient food be placed in the trough that the weaners will eat in 10 minutes. If the trough is cleaned up within 10 minutes, at the next feed, increase volume by 20 %.

Place dry creep feed in the normal feeders by hand.

3 Repeat step 2 at 2 hour intervals.

If weaners are not eating

Note and mark all weaners who shy away from the trough and refuse to eat at the first 2 occasions.

At the 3rd time pick up all the weaners who have refused to eat. Place the weaner by the feed trough and encourage, using fingers if necessary, the weaner to eat.

4 At the end of the first day of weaning: after the 3rd feeding opportunity is finished, turn off the lights to encourage the weaners to sleep.

Second day

1 Feed gruel to the pigs every 2 hours. Therefore, feed 6 times per day.

2 Note the increases in volume and dryness of the feed.

3 At the end of the day, switch off the lights again and allow the pigs to sleep.

The feeding interval is intended to prevent the weaners from screaming after their lost mothers.

4 Increase the amount of feed in the normal feeders – still fed by hand.

Third day

1. Continue feeding gruel and extend the feeding interval to every 3 hours – therefore 4 times per day.

2. Turn on normal creep feeders.

Fourth day

1. Feed only one gruel 2 hours after daybreak. Observe the weaners' behaviour. If the pigs are well settled, no further manual feeding is required.

2. Ensure normal feeders are working and adjusted as normally required.

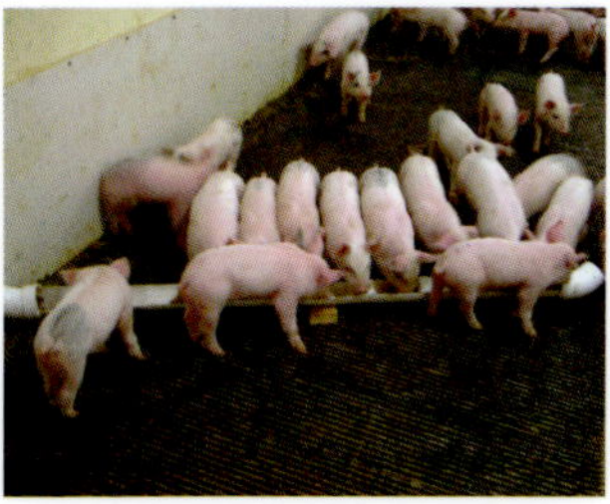

Weaners eating out of a trough feeder.

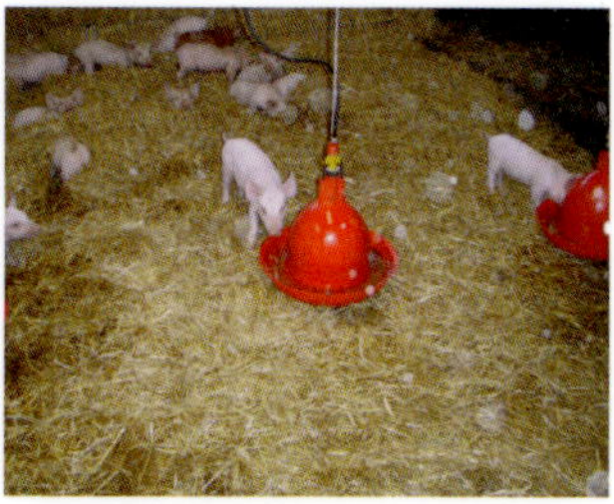

Turkey drinkers may be useful at the beginning of growing.

Caring for the lower order pigs

If the bottom 10 % of pigs at weaning are streamed into a separate environment, it is possible to modify the gruel-feeding programme to cover 7 days, rather than the 3 days proscribed.

> Note, however, it is essential to get the pig's eating normal creep feed as soon as possible, otherwise a "double weaning" event will occur, which will put the pig's back significantly.

Disadvantages or problems

If gruel feeding is continued too long a double weaning event will occur. The gruel feed costs a lot of money and it is essential it is only used to ensure all the weaned pigs learn to eat normal quantities of creep feed post-weaning.

If diarrhoea starts check product quality and reduce the interval of feedings.

If pigs do not eat up the volume within 10 minutes, reduce next feed volume by 10 %.

If there is too much food provided you are cheating on the human time element – resulting in a loss of the weaner's normal behaviour.

None talkative stockpeople do not mimic the sow's normal calling behaviour.

Why put this much effort into the first 5 days post-weaning?

- To reduce the incidence of post-weaning ill-thrift.
- Reduce post-weaning diarrhoea: weaners who fail to eat properly, will gorge when they start to eat and diarrhoea occurs 2 days later.
- To enhance the growth of the pigs to finish. Good feed intake (> 250 g/day) in the first week is worth over 10 days to finish at 110 kg liveweight.

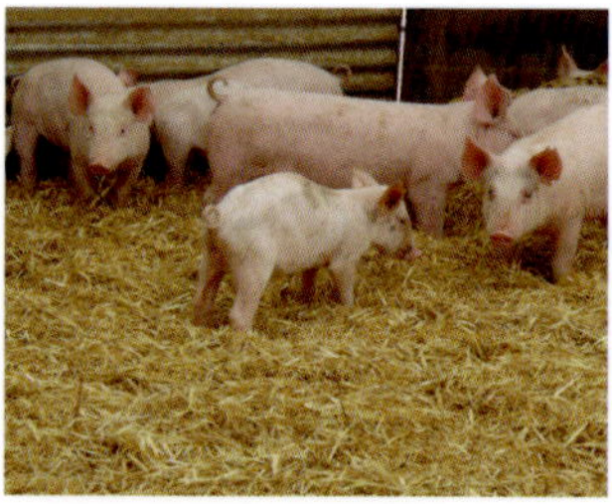

Ill-thrift in a weaner - starved.

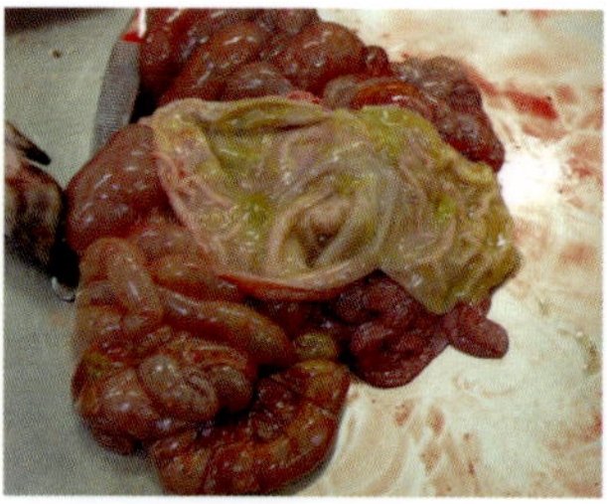

Empty stomach and intestines.

APP – *Actinobacillus pleuropneumoniae* investigation

Undisturbed group of pigs	Examine and record lying pattern of undisturbed pigs – picture/video.
	Behaviour of pigs around the water supply – picture/video.
	Behaviour of pigs around the feeders – picture/video.
Stock	Clinical pigs respond to tulathromycin, ceftiofur, penicillin.
	Is Tilmicosin used in – feed or water medication?
	Record post – weaning antibiotic use.
	Is any APP vaccine used?
Check for PRRSv	Blood results – note 21 days antibody delay.
PMWS/PCVAD	Were pigs vaccinated against PCV2 at weaning?
	Check vaccine purchases correspond to weaning numbers.
	Check medicine storage (2-8 °C).
Post-mortem	Ensure diagnosis correct - picture/video.
	Has APP actually being isolated? Type of APP isolated.
	Slaughterhouse reports.
Sick pigs	Treatment of sick pigs.
	Movement of recovered pigs.
	Collect true mortality and morbidity figures.
Check weaning age and weight	Age at weaning.
	Weight at weaning.
Immunology	Feedback programme.
Pig flow	Collect true weaning/farrowing/breeding and gilt numbers by batch.
All-in/all-out	AIAO by pigs, water, feed, floor, air and medicine.

Continued ▸

Medicines	Ensure needles and syringes not used between different batches.
Water	Flow suitable for the pigs.
	Height suitable for the pigs.
	Number of drinkers.
	Cleaning programme between batches.
Floor	Stocking density.
	Cleaning programme between batches.
Air	Temperature variation.
	Relative humidity (50-75 % RH).
	High dust and endotoxin issues.
	Note level of slurry under slats how is the air flow from underneath slats?
	Draughts in the proposed sleeping area.
	Examine defecation pattern of pigs.
	Smoke buildings and record air movement patterns- picture/video.
	Cleaning programme between batches.
Feed	Feed space and feeder management.
	Problem coincides with a change in diet/feed type and feed size.
	Cleaning programme between batches.
Other problems	PRRSv, PCVAD/PMWS and mange are classical examples of problems.
	Eliminate any additional stressors– weighing, tagging, bleeding.

Review "*The basic stockmanship guide: Pigs, Hogs and Swine*" (John Carr, Editorial Servet, 2013).

Medication marks

One way to get our pigs to talk to us is to use stockmanship marks effectively, so that the whole farm health team know what is going on. We all mark our pigs with spray markers to indicate which are in heat or which we have treated. But can we use these marks in different ways to transmit more information. We present four stockmanship ideas to illustrate this concept.

Number of times the pig has been treated

Most injections are either one day or three day treatments. The three day treatment options are the most difficult to ensure compliance especially over the weekend, when different staff may be doing the treatment. Placing the treatment mark in different positions around the body can help inform the whole team.

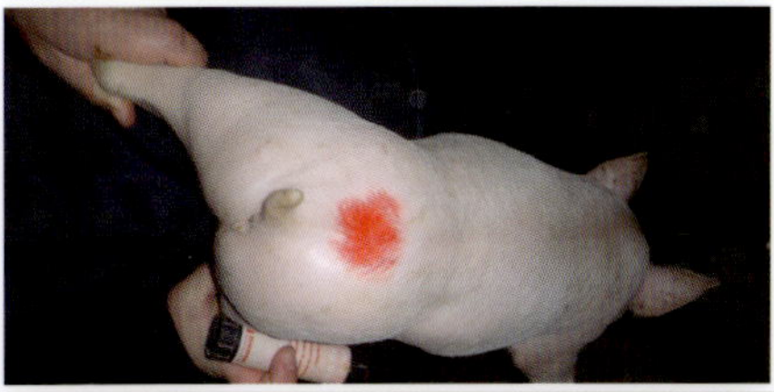

Day 1

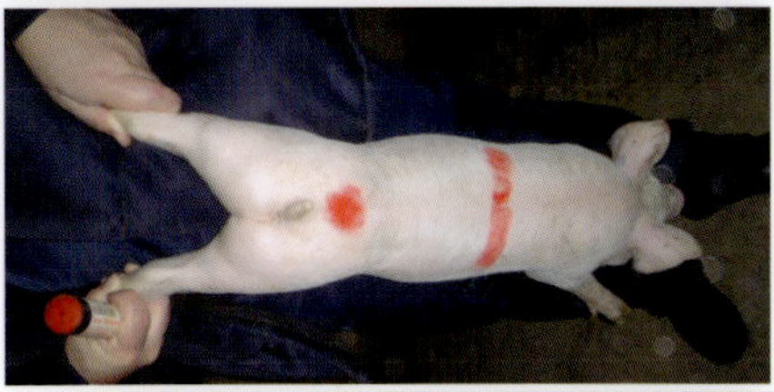

Day 2

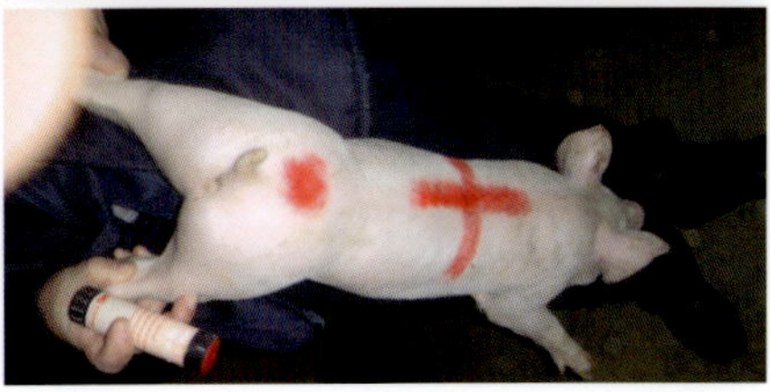

Day 3

What was the pig treated for?

This can be particularly useful in the farrowing house. Marking the piglet in well co-ordinated patterns can tell the whole team why the pig was treated.

Mark on rump – scouring

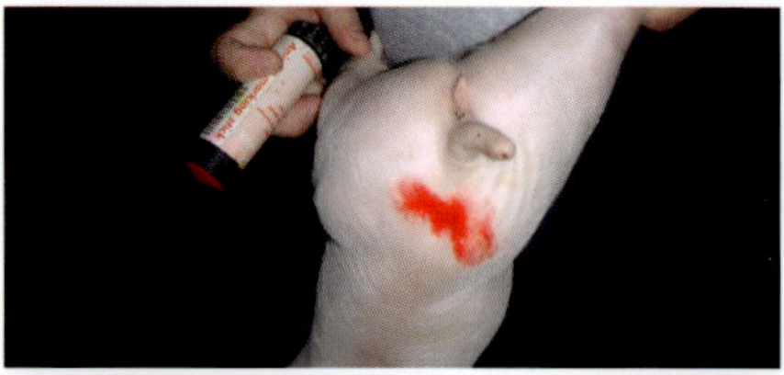

Mark on arm or leg – lame on that leg (right fore limb in this example)

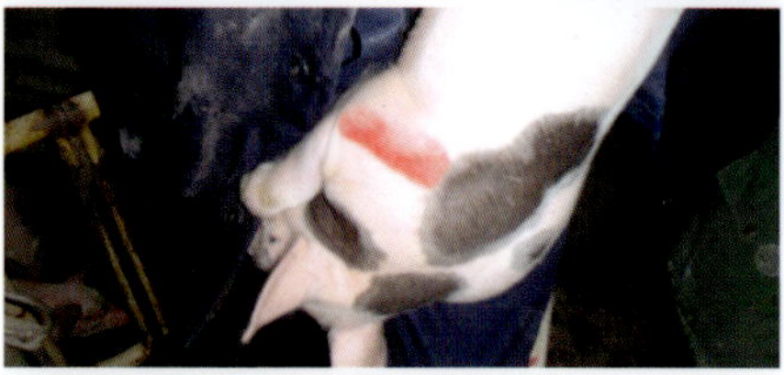

Mark along back – chest issue – pneumonia

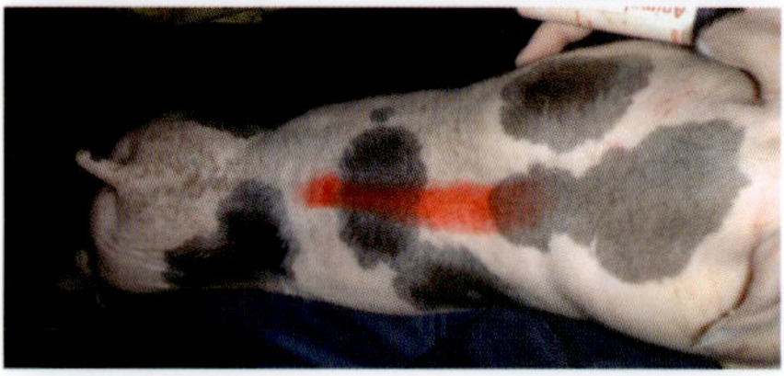

Mark on head – facial necrosis or meningitis

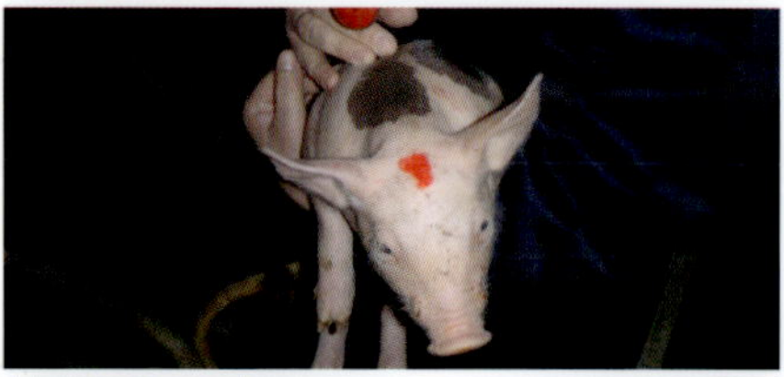

Mark across back – problem underneath (e.g. umbilical abscess)

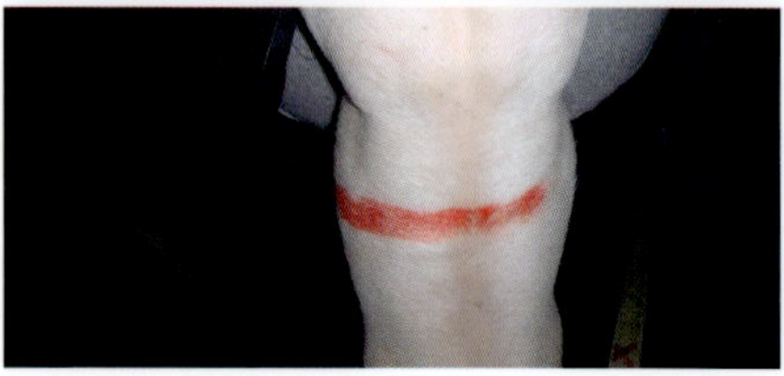

This can then be combined with different colours to indicate different treatment products.

When are the weaned sows going to come back into heat?

A lot of useful information gets lost between the farrowing and breeding. A major predictor of the wean to service interval is the appetite during lactation.

Sows who eat poorly during lactation are most likely to have a delayed weaned to service interval. So get the breeding guys to mark these sows while they are in still their farrowing place – day before weaning for example.

Then place these sows in their own group at the end of the breeding row. Obviously check them from day 4 post-weaning, but do not be surprised when they are actually only having a short heat on day 7! Obviously if you have reached your breeding target these might become cull sows anyway.

The second group which is going to have an extra day with their wean-to-service period is the 1st parity sows (gilt litter). All these sows should be marked as placed at the end of the breeding row.

How long do marks last?

One downside of marks is that they do not last long! One trick around this is to trim the hair instead of using a paint stick marker – this will last 2 weeks at least – and is cheap!

> But do not over do these marks – it can become extremely confusing both for the stockpeople and perhaps the sow's friends?

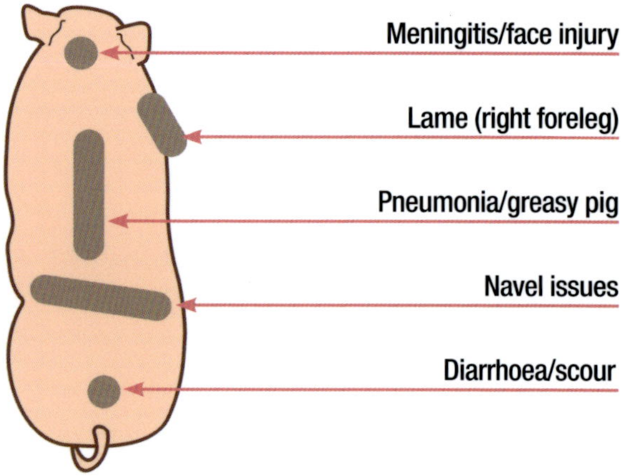

Hospital pen design

1 Deep dry straw bedding covering a non-slip, insulated concrete floor.

2 Good draught free ventilation. The provision of a kennelled area should be available.

3 Provide an individual feeder, which is hand filled twice daily. There should never be a lot of food in the feeders so that in-feed medication is possible.

4 Provide a bowl drinker which is set at 30 cm above the ground for 20 kg pigs or more. This drinker should be fed from a separate header tank to enable easy medication if necessary.

5 Easy entry and exit points which do not necessitate lifting of the animal over steps.

6 Pigs in this pen should be examined a minimum of twice daily and the hospital pen records should be completed.

7 All hospital pen pigs should be tagged and treated as individuals on entry.

8 Pigs in the sick pen may need a companion.

9 Each hospital pen should be of adequate size to hold up to ten pigs.

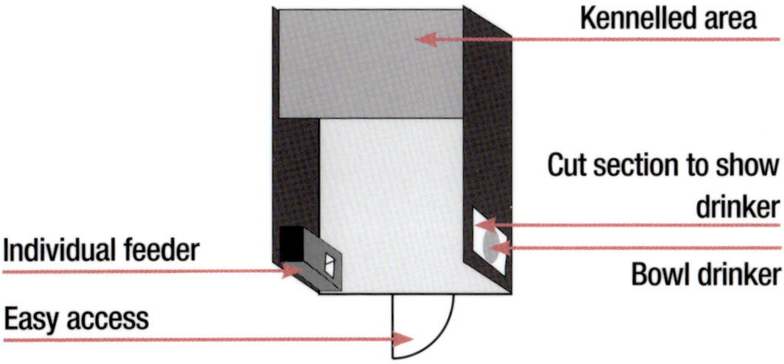

Factors affecting the yield of pig meat

Breeding programme

The single most important reason why insufficient quantities of meat is sold per week, per square metre of finishing floor is related to insufficient sows/gilts being served some 6 months previously. Adaptation to known times of reduced farrowing rate or litter size, this must be accommodated by the breeding or more females.

The aim must be to fill a truck.

Growth rate and feed intake

Any factor which will reduce the feed intake or growth rate will reduce the farm yield. These include overstocking, poor feed troughs, marginal water supplies, poor temperature controls, poor air quality.

Single-sex feeding.

Contact with the abattoir/abattoirs (major customers)

Close liaison with abattoir to determine exactly what type of meat they require. There will be only a few customers in your area, determine what they want.

Possibly use thirst-making feeds at end.

Slaughter at the correct weight

Supplying pigs that are less variable in the slaughterhouse, this may require twice-weekly shipping.

Shipping closer to the maximum permitted weight.

Calculate the relative cost of 5 % overweights, as compared with 5 % underweight.

Negotiate a higher weight contract; however, ensure that the contract then does not become attractive to other suppliers.

Use a weigh scale regularly. Check the weigh scale at least monthly with standardised weights, not your own, variable weight.

Monitor growth rates for each week. Weigh all pigs when you have to move them – weaning, out of the nursery at slaughter.

Correct conformation and lean tissue content, P_2 measurement

Require that the genetic make-up matches customers demand with a move towards blocky compact.

Genetics. Use meat-type sires.

Correct matching of feed to genetic potential.

Correct environment to allow fulfilment of genetic potential.

Taking advantage of any premium markets, i.e. welfare contract note requirements of piglet processing/housing.

Slaughtering

The journey time to slaughterhouse should be short. Stress free as possible journey, note stocking density, quality of roads (including your own drive), journey plan.

Known slaughter time. Last feed 12 hours before killing. Lairage water available both for drinking and cooling.

Killing must be do promptly.

Post-weaning diseases

Effective health maintenance programmes.

Attention to suppressing 'nutritional' scours post-weaning.

Effective and prompt treatment of compromised pigs to reduce chronic ill thrift pigs, which may end up condemned anyway.

> Moving the average dead weight by 1 kg (say 79 to 80 kg) is worth 2700 kg per 100 sows doing 27 pigs per sow per year.

The aim is to produce a highly desirable quality product time and time again.

World meat consumption 2006 (FAO)

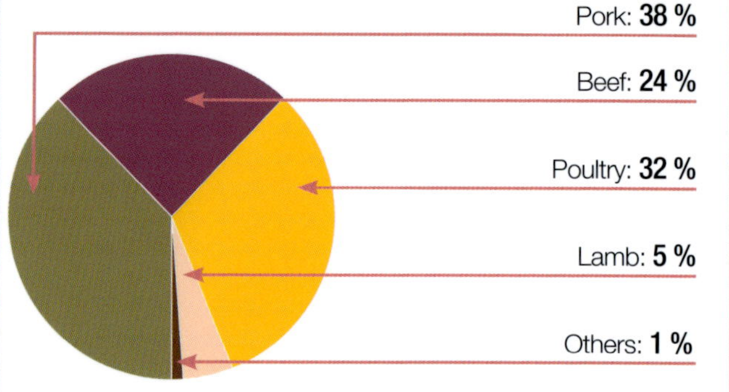

What is the P_2 measurement?

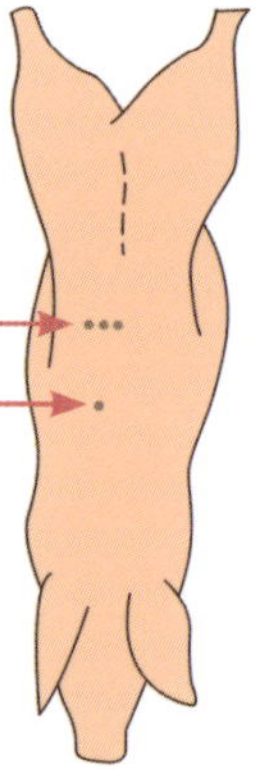

P_1, P_2 and P_3 locations

Rib fat location

P_1, P_2 and P_3 have to be taken level with the head of the last rib.

Rib fat taken 6 cm from the dorsal mid-line between the 3rd and 4th last rib.

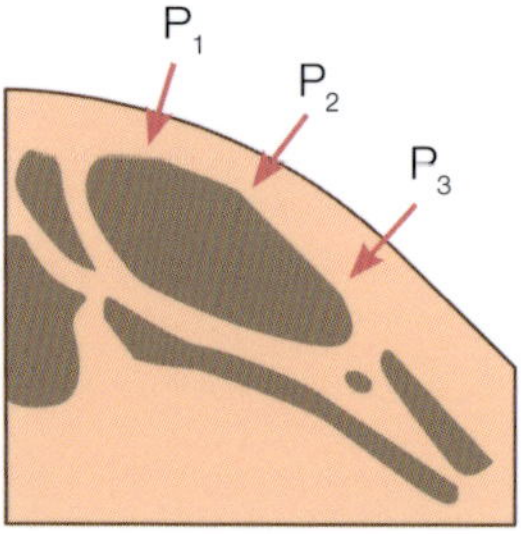

The P_1 measurement is taken 4.5 cm from midline.

The P_2 measurement is taken 6.5 cm from midline.

The P_3 measurement is taken 8.0 cm from midline.

Lean meat percentage and EU grades:

- S 60 % or more
- E 55 – 59 %
- U 50 – 54 %
- R 45 – 49 %
- O 40 – 44 %
- P less than 40 %

Lean composition is protein 23 %, fat 2 % and water 75 %.

Factors that can affect meat quality

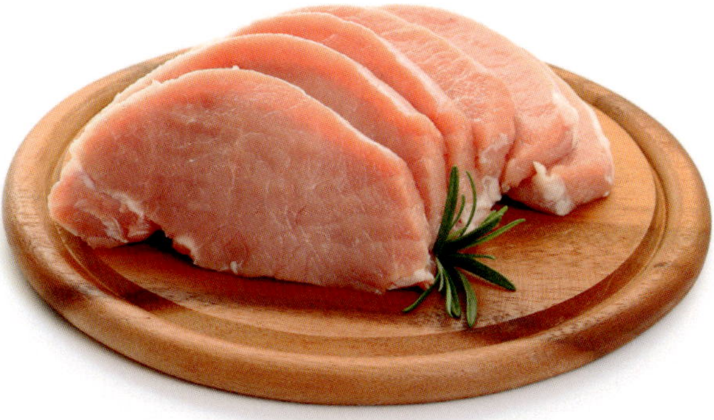

- Lairage time
- Lairage conditions
- Animal handling
- Transport
- Diseases
- Slaughter weight
- Climate
- Genetics
- Nutrition
- Social environment
- Cooking
- Ageing time
- Post-slaughter handling
- pH at 24 hours (ideally 5.8)
- Slaughter procedure
- Pre-slaughter handling

Dead-weight to live-weight

Dead-weight to live-weight (kg)

Dead weight	Live weight	Dead weight	Live weight	Dead weight	Live weight
32	45.5	55	75	78	105
33	46.5	56	76.5	79	106
34	48	57	78	80	107.5
35	49	58	79.5	81	109
36	50.5	59	80.5	82	110
37	52	60	82.5	83	111
38	53.5	61	84	84	112
39	55	62	85	85	113
40	56.5	63	86	86	114
41	58	64	87	87	115
42	59.5	65	88	88	115.5
43	60.5	66	89	89	116.5
44	61.5	67	90.5	90	117.5
45	63	68	92	91	118.5
46	64.5	69	93	92	119
47	66	70	94.5	93	120
48	67.5	71	96	94	120.5
49	69	72	97.5	95	121.5
50	70	73	99	96	122.5
51	71	74	100	97	123
52	72	75	101.5	98	124
53	73.5	76	103	99	124.5
54	74.5	77	104	100	125

Greenhouse carbon footprint on animals

Carbon footprint is the intensity of some common foods expressed as kg of carbon dioxide-equivalent (CO_2-e) released into the atmosphere for each kg of production.

For foods that produce copious amounts of methane, the 20-year figures are substantially higher than over a 100-year time frame.

Food	kg CO_2-e/kg (20 years)	kg CO_2-e/kg (100 years)	Scientific American Feb 2009 (kg/year)
Beef meat	111.1	55.5	14.50
Sheep meat and wool	96.3	32.7	-
Pig meat	10.5	3.5	3.8
Rice	2.4	0.74	-
Poultry meat	1.3	0.38	1.1
Wheat	0.35	0.32	-
Potatoes	-	-	0.26
Apples	-	-	0.3
Asparagus	-	-	0.52

Manager's weekly report

Date...

Area	1	2	3
Needle security			
Medicine storage			
Foot bath hygiene			
Boot hygiene			
Farrowing area			
• Hygiene			
• Water			
• Feed			
• Floor			
• Ventilation			
• Stock - sows			
• Stock - piglets			
Sow & gilt house			
• Hygiene			
• Water			
• Feed			
• Floor			
• Ventilation			
• Stock - sows			
• Stock - gilts			
• Stock - boars			
First stage nursery			
• Hygiene			
• Water			
• Feed			
• Floor			
• Ventilation			
• Stock			

Area	1	2	3
Second stage nursery			
• Hygiene			
• Water			
• Feed			
• Floor			
• Ventilation			
• Stock			
Grower house			
• Hygiene			
• Water			
• Feed			
• Floor			
• Ventilation			
• Stock			
Finisher house			
• Hygiene			
• Water			
• Feed			
• Floor			
• Ventilation			
• Stock			
Loading area			
Gilt isolation			
Artificial insemination laboratory			
Staff canteen			
External appearance			
Teeth clippers			
Tail docker			
Slap marker			

Interpretation of scores
3: Good; 2: Attention to detail needed; 1: Room for improvement

Signed: ....

Management timetable

Monday weaning (2-3 hours daily).

Monday afternoon

Major event: weaning day.

Nursery

Review weaned pigs, in particular selection and distribution of pigs. Are there pigs to euthanise?

Is staff prepared to feed and look after newly weaned pigs?

Service area

Review gilt pool selection for the next batch breeding.

Tuesday afternoon

Major events: routine weekly check.

General review

Walk farm with area manager and complete management record; in particular review newly weaned pigs. Have all weaned pigs eaten?

Review farrowing house cleaning programme.

Review medicine, needle, syringe hygiene.

Wednesday afternoon

Major events: farrowing house set up + grow/finish review.

Farrowing house

Examine farrowing house with newly entered sows. Was room set up adequately? All drinkers work? Is staff prepared for sows to farrow?

Grow/finish

Walk along the grow/finish barn, in particular check all feeders for wasted feed.

Check if drinkers work.

Check the ventilation system – review draughts in particular.

Hospital/compromised pig pens.

Are there pigs to euthanise?

Ensure AI semen coming on Thursday afternoon.

Friday/Saturday

Major events: services.

Service area

Review and observe breeding routines.

Are sufficient sows/gilts available to meet batch service targets?

Review gilt requirements in 9-10 weeks time.

Sunday

Major event: service/weaner accommodation.

Service area

Review and observe breeding routines.

Nursery

Review hygiene/cleaning standards of the nursery. Are they prepared for the next batch of newly weaned pigs?

The above programme is designed for a weekly batch system.

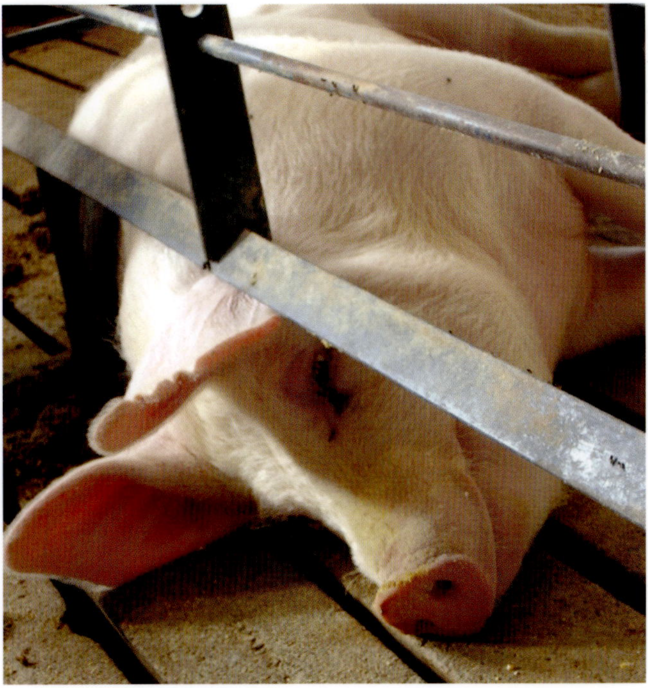